WEIGHT LOSS
Tathastu

Learn How Not to Lose Your Weight the Wrong Way

BHUSHAN GAONKAR

FOUNDER - FITNESSMESSENGERS

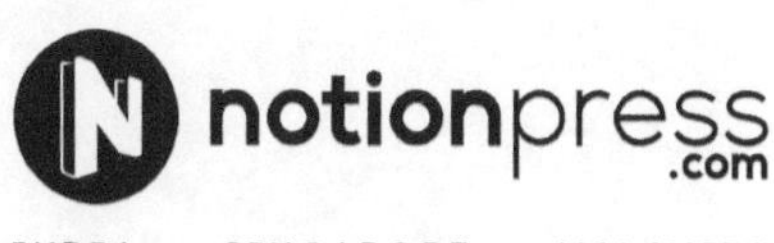

notionpress.com

INDIA • SINGAPORE • MALAYSIA

Notion Press

No.8, 3rd Cross Street,
CIT Colony, Mylapore,
Chennai, Tamil Nadu – 600004

First Published by Notion Press 2021
Copyright © Bhushan Gaonkar 2021
All Rights Reserved.

ISBN 978-1-63806-684-2

Disclaimer

Please consult your doctor before starting an exercise programme, especially if you haven't exercised before or haven't exercised in the last six months. While exercising, if you feel any pain or discomfort, please check with your doctor.

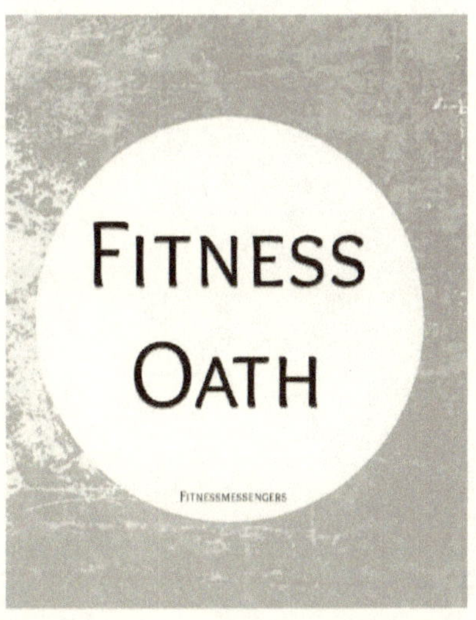

Hola Friends, let us take a Fitness Oath.

"I aspire to be fit and will make the required efforts, consistently."

Sign here, put today's date, and let the world know about it.

____

Fitnessmessengers

Contents

Synopsis   9

About the Author   19

Chapter 1   Current Scenario   23

Chapter 2   Break The Barriers   33

Chapter 3   Think Beyond Scale   58

Chapter 4   How to Start   66

Chapter 5   Self-Assessment   73

Chapter 6   Setting Fitness Goals   78

Chapter 7   Exercise to Get Stronger   88

Chapter 8   Managing Your Meals   126

Chapter 9   Do You Have Cheat Meals?   154

Chapter 10   Managing Social Events   158

Chapter 11   How Good Is Your Digestion?   165

Chapter 12   Let's Shop the Right Way.   175

Chapter 13   Read the Label   183

Chapter 14   Do You Cook Right?   188

Contents

Chapter 15 Do You Have Sweet Tooth?   199

Chapter 16 Let's Break a Few Fitness Myths   205

Chapter 17 Fitness Lifestyle   217

Chapter 18 No More Broken Hearts   230

Chapter 19 For The Records   233

Chapter 20 Do You Switch Off?   238

Chapter 21 Stress   249

Chapter 22 Child Obesity   255

Chapter 23 What Next?   263

How Fitness Changed My Life: By Coach Anagha   267

Appendix and Resources   275

Acknowledgements   279

Synopsis

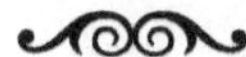

Ashwika is a young mother and works in a financial organisation. We were discussing how two of her colleagues had lost weight by following some diet and how keen she was to get fit, so she could play with her kid.

Ashwika: I am a foodie and cannot diet! Can you still help me get fit?

Me: You don't need to diet to get fit! You need a good lifestyle.

Ashwika: What do you mean?

Me: You need to build good eating habits and be active.

Ashwika: Will doing just this help?

Me: Only this will help you.

Ashwika: How much time will it take?

Me: It depends on how soon you can adapt and follow.

Ashwika: But I can't give up on rice and roti, that's my staple.

Me: You need not, in fact, it should be an essential part of your meals

Ashwika: But isn't rice fattening? And gluten is bad for health?

Me: Absolutely not, they are a good source of energy.

Me: Are you gluten intolerant?

Ashwika: I don't know, but my colleagues who have lost weight have given up roti and rice completely.

Me: But do they crave rice when you have lunch at the office?

Ashwika: Yes, they do, but then they control their cravings.

Me: So, what do they eat?

Ashwika: They don't eat much, mostly salads, juices, and crackers.

Me: Can you eat like them?

Ashwika: No

Me: But they have lost weight, and you too want to shed some kilos!

Ashwika: I can't eat like them; I want to enjoy my meals.

Me: Do they exercise regularly?

Ashwika: They walk a lot.

Me: Do they look strong?

Ashwika: No

Me: Do you want to eat your favourite foods, get strong, and still enjoy the journey?

Ashwika: I would love to, is it possible?

Me: Absolutely!

Ashwika: Let's do it then.

This is a typical conversation with most of my clients.

The common misconception I notice in all these conversations is the belief that one must diet to get fit.

Anyone who wants to get fit just follows these rules mindlessly:

Don't eat rice.

Eat only salads.

Banana is fattening.

Have only olive oil.

Walk for 90 minutes a day.

Skip your dinner.

Have detox water.

Some do get results in terms of weight loss by following such practices, but ask yourself:

Is it sustainable? Can you be on a diet for ages?

No, right!

This book is conceptualised to give the following message: You don't need a magical diet to get fit, you need to build a good lifestyle. This message is elucidated by real-life examples and practical tips.

I am not the first and surely not the last person to write about this issue. Some amazing authors have written about it. Then what is different about my book?

Concepts do not change much; I have correlated these concepts with real-life examples, having worked with different people. Throughout the book, there are tips that have been tried and tested on many, including me, my family, and the people I have worked with, wherein I have seen fantastic and sustainable results.

Everyone wants to get fit and look good, why would anyone not? I have spoken to young mothers, working professionals, housewives, teens, people facing obesity issues, who struggle with their fitness.

It's not that people are not making any effort to get fit, but there are limitations in terms of time, money, awareness, etc. And it involves so much more than just diet and exercise. Hence, I have included the chapter *Break The Barriers*, which identifies the common barriers and suggests tips that can help you overcome them. For example, one of the common barriers is lack of motivation, and practising this simple tip can help you overcome it:

Extract from Chapter 2: Break the barriers

I do not have the motivation to work on my fitness, how do I start?

Try this trick:

Old clothes trial: It's time to clean the wardrobe and locate your favourite old shirt or a pair of jeans which you loved wearing to college/office but you no longer wear it as you can't fit into it.

Go back to the lovely memories you had wearing it. It may be your first date, or your best friend's wedding, or a successful job interview.

Next, wash and iron it and keep it in your clothes rack, such that every time you open the rack, it's visible.

When you start seeing it daily, you will think about all the good memories associated with it and want to fit into it again. When this process happens daily for weeks together, there are high chances that the nostalgic feelings will push you to do something about your health and you may actually start exercising just to fit into your favourite clothes.

Do consider any start as a good start.

Doing this is not difficult and if it helps you get started, then there's nothing like it. Similarly, there are more such examples throughout the book.

Another thing which I have seen is whenever one wants to get fit, they start walking or running, with no focus on strength training. There is a lack of awareness around strength training and the long-term benefit it offers. More than awareness, there are myths around it, which keeps people away from it. Strength training will make me look bulky, it's only for bodybuilders, etc. I have a chapter dedicated to this area and have tried to explain it in the best possible way.

To give you a better idea of what I have covered in this book, please have a look at the below section.

How this book is structured?

It has multiple chapters and I have tried putting them in a logical sequence which will allow readers to practically implement the lessons.

Chapter 1 throws light on the current scenario regarding health and fitness, where I have highlighted the sedentary lifestyle of people and the problems it has created.

Chapter 2 is all about breaking the barriers and getting started on your fitness journey. Generally, people want to get fit, but then there are practical problems that come in the way. This chapter will focus on giving solutions to the most common barriers.

Chapter 3 will make you think about real fitness. Is it only weight loss or are there other important parameters too?

Chapter 4 is about initiating your fitness journey. Here, we give you a peek at Ketaki's real transformation and how she managed to get fit by shedding her post-maternity weight. This is an inspiring story.

Chapter 5 is about self-assessment, understanding your current state of fitness. Here, you will find quantifiable ways to measure your fitness parameters that will help identify a starting point.

Chapter 6 is about setting your fitness goals. This is where you become serious about your fitness and start making plans for it. Goals provide the right direction and motivate us when things don't go as per plan.

Chapter 7 is about exercise and doing it the right way. In fact, there are more wrong ways to exercise than you can think of and it can actually reverse the benefits. There is so much more to know about exercise than just sweating it out in the gym, right from what you eat and how to manage injuries.

Chapter 8 is all about eating the right foods. What and when you eat influences your fitness more than anything else. Here, we discuss planning meals and nutrition along with other essential parameters.

Chapter 9 will show you how to have cheat meals, not literally! You would have heard that people have lost weight even after eating ice cream! This chapter will motivate you to eat your favourite foods and still stay healthy.

Chapter 10 is about managing social events. Our fitness journey can't be restricted to exercise and eating right. We have friends and families and there are events too. Just because one has decided to get fit, he/she cannot always avoid parties and celebrations. This chapter highlights a few best practices which help you enjoy your social life too.

Chapter 11 deals with another important aspect of fitness: Digestion. You may eat the best foods, but if your digestion is not good, then your body doesn't get any benefit. We also talk about how constipation has become a universal problem and how you can deal with it. The role of water is also highlighted here.

Chapter 12 is interesting as it talks about food shopping. With a plethora of options available, how does one make the right choice? I've listed a few tips to make shopping for food and groceries a healthy experience.

Chapter 13 will show you how to read food labels. With the mall culture growing at a rapid pace, the health food market has expanded in no time and the consumer is spoilt for choice. Reading labels will help you make informed decisions, in line with your fitness goals.

Chapter 14 is about simple tips on cooking the right way. The best ingredients will not help if they are not cooked the right way. Right from cooking on high flame, to the usage of oils, sauces, and spices, everything matters.

Chapter 15 deals with sugar and how it impacts our health. People talk about sweet cravings post meals. In this chapter, we find ways to minimise them. And it's not just about white sugar, but also about foods that contain sugar.

Chapter 16 is a myth breaker. For ages, we have been following certain myths and it makes sense to look at them with a wider lens. I have taken the most common ones and put forward my perspective to help you make the right decision.

Chapter 17 highlights the importance of a healthy lifestyle which is a precursor to long-term fitness. There are ways to stay fit even after you have met your fitness goals.

Chapter 18 is all about the heart and how exercise can help you strengthen it. We talk about a few dos and don'ts to take care of your heart.

Chapter 19 will show you how to keep records of your exercise and meal plans. It helps you introspect when things don't go as planned.

Chapter 20 talks about the importance of sleep and how one can sleep better. I have established a relationship between sleep and fat loss and have added tips that will help you improve the quality of sleep. Common distractors to sleep are also discussed and ways to manage them are mentioned.

Chapter 21 focuses on mental fitness and emphasises the fact that stress can make one obese. Your fitness journey can be an emotional process and you need to be strong enough to manage it. I have added a few tips which can help you do this.

Chapter 22 is very important from the perspective of future generations. Child obesity is on the rise and it is our responsibility as parents and elders to show them the right way, not just by telling them to be active and eating right, but by following the same also. I have mentioned a few tips which can help kids resort to a healthy lifestyle.

Chapter 23 is the last chapter, which emphasises just one thing: Initiate your journey by taking the first step. It feels good to read success stories, but it's equally important to create one. This chapter also offers a bird's eye view of all the concepts discussed in this book.

There is an appendix section that has many resources like exercise videos, a video on muscle meditation, warm-ups and stretching videos, which can be referred to and added to your exercise schedule.

I have also added the transformation journey of coach Anagha.

Additionally, it has more information about our services, right from functional training to transformation programmes for individuals and organisations.

I welcome you onboard this amazing journey and am sure you will have a great one. For any queries, feel free to connect with me at fitnessmessengers@gmail.com.

Thanks,

Bhushan Gaonkar,

Fitnessmessengers.

About the Author

An IT professional who wants to stay fit.

Hello Everybody,

I am Bhushan and I feel great about writing this book. Doing a desk job for more than 15 years now, I understand the sedentary nature of many other working professionals. Nine to ten hours of work and another one to two hours of travel consumes almost 50 per cent of your time. Then there are other things to do too, household work, family commitments, social life, etc. To fit all this in 24 hours and still find time for fitness is a challenge for many.

Isn't it?

I would say Yes and a No.

I started exercising much before I started working, right from my college days. So, it had become a part of my routine or what I call my lifestyle.

And when I started working, I just made time for it.

Were there any changes to my routine?

Yes, the workout sessions were reduced to 30 minutes, unlike the earlier 60–90 minutes.

The frequency came down to four days a week from six. That's it.

I realised early in my career that our working commitments are not a showstopper to get fit. It is our mindset which creates an impression that we are busy.

Tell me when were we the fittest?

I think when we were kids.

Do you think kids are not tied up? Just look at their routine.

Long school hours, assignments, projects, tests, exams, coaching classes, and on top of that, trying to meet parents' expectations.

Sometimes I feel my kid is busier than me.

But I still find him jumping around from one room to another.

So, it is not about time, it is about how we manage it, making fitness a priority.

And how do we do it?

The solution is to make fitness part of our routine, so it does not create an impression that we are doing something unnecessary. The way we brush our teeth daily without any reminders, we can exercise and eat well too.

Why do we need reminders for this?

The next question everybody may ask is:

How do we make fitness a part of our lifestyle?

This book is all about answering this question.

Happy reading.

About Fitnessmessengers

Fitness Messengers (Fitnessmessengers) is a fitness-motivation initiative focused on changing people's lives by making simple and sustainable lifestyle changes.

We are a team of Wellness coaches focusing on exercise, nutrition, and meal management and each of us has gone through the cycle of transforming our body, hence we understand the science and the emotions behind it.

We facilitate these transformations by inculcating the habits of exercising and eating right. We also believe that wellness is a long-term goal. It's not just temporary weight loss or weight gain done through crash diets. Thus, we educate our participants to help them understand the basics of fitness and its relation to the right nutrition and an active lifestyle.

To know about our offerings on Workouts, Employee Wellness Programmes, Get Fit workshops, Body Transformation, visit our website: http://fitnessmessengers.com/Service.aspx

Chapter 1
Current Scenario

It was around 6:30 p.m. on a Friday. I had just finished dinner and was surfing through channels on my smart TV (actually dumb) when I got a call from a 24-year-old Rushabh.

Rushabh: Hello, do you offer a weight loss programme?

Me: Yes, we do body transformations by focusing on exercise and eating right. What are you looking for?

Rushabh: I want to lose weight.

Me: We will help you lose fat, which will eventually reduce your weight.

Rushabh: How much time will it take?

Me: It depends on multiple factors.

Rushabh: Yes, of course. I will not miss an exercise session, give up rice and bread and drink five to six cups of green tea for the next two months. Will I lose 15 kgs?

I could sense the desperation.

Me: Hold on Rushabh, such a stringent timeline will not work. We need to understand your lifestyle, put you through the exercise sessions, set up a meal guideline, check on how you adapt to it and make corrections as needed. This is what it's going to take. It also depends on how consistently you follow it, not just for one or two weeks.

He was taken aback listening to what I had said.

Rushabh: This means I cannot look fit in the next two months? My college friend lost 22 kgs in three and a half months and I also hope to do the same.

Me: I don't know your lifestyle, so telling you something which I am not sure of will not make sense. Why don't you tell me more about yourself?

Rushabh: I want to lose weight and for this, I am ready to do whatever you tell me to do.

Me: As per the process, I will share a fitness questionnaire with you. Get back to me with your details and then let us connect on a video call at 8:00 p.m. today.

He said he would give me the details quickly and we fixed the 8:00 p.m. call the same day.

Our fitness questionnaire is a detailed one. It helps us understand the customer in the right way to make an action plan. I received his details and was surprised on reading his daily routine:

> *Rushabh's routine:*
>
> GM: 8 am
>
> First Meal: 8:45 – Black coffee
>
> 10:00 am – Tea and few biscuits
>
> 11:15 am – Tea (cutting)
>
> 2:30 pm – Lunch (Puri bhaji/Fried rice/Pav bhaji/Maggi/ Tava Pulav)
>
> 3:00 pm – Tea (cutting)
>
> 6:00 pm – Tea (cutting)
>
> 7:30–8:00 pm – Sandwich/Samosa/Bhel/Wada Pav + Tea (cutting)
>
> 10:30–11:00 pm – Dinner (Chapati-bhaji + Dal-Rice/Dal-Khicdi)
>
> 12:00 am – On bed with Web series and Social Media
>
> 2.00–2:30 am – GN

A couple of things I could highlight immediately:

- Heavy consumption of tea throughout the day (read TEA as SUGAR)
- Very late dinner

But a detailed look revealed more:

- He started his day with a dose of caffeine.
- His next meal was tea and biscuits.
- **His actual first meal was at 2:30 p.m.**, that too not a healthy meal.

- He consumed a lot of junk/fried food daily.

- Of course, a very late and heavy dinner is sinful.

- He slept very late and not for more than six hours.

Based on his info, I made quick notes and discussed them with him. He patiently listened to all I had to say:

Rushabh: I will follow everything and eat whatever and whenever you say, provided you assure me that I will lose weight.

Me: Let me explain where you are going wrong.

Your body doesn't get energy while you sleep, so you must give it the right nutrition as soon as you get up. That's why it's called breakfast (break – your – fast).

Not sure whether this is true, but this is what I tell most of my customers.

You have been having tea-coffee-biscuits as your first meal, which does not give the right nutrition to your body, pushing it into starvation and craving mode.

Second, what you have been eating for lunch has no nutrition at all, though it takes care of your hunger. The way your luxury car cannot run on kerosene (even though it's a fuel), your body cannot function effectively on these junk foods.

As I spoke, he nodded his head. It was a video call, so I could see that. I prefer video calls or face to face discussions, so I can sense body language. In fact, it gives me a hint as to whether the person will commit to it seriously.

Third, the cups of tea you sip throughout the day are adding to your problems.

Rushabh: I take only half a cup or cutting (as it is called)…it's just three to four sips.

Me: With every glass and every sip, you are adding sugar to your body, which is one of the main reasons you are gaining weight (fat).

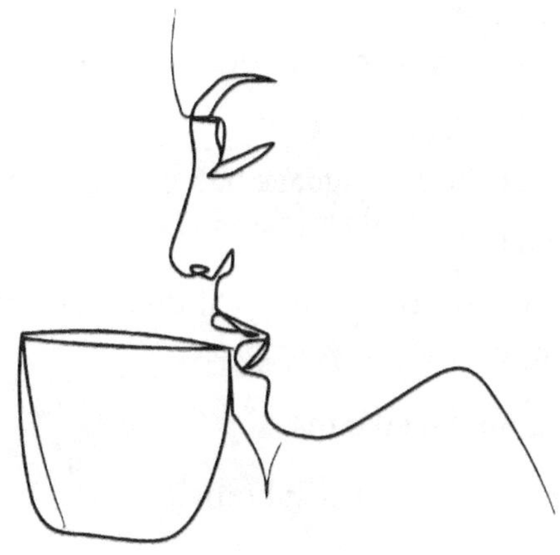

I think it was a moment of happy realisation for him.

Me: Fourth, there is a big gap between your lunch and the next meal.

Rushabh: I do not feel hungry, so how can I eat?

Me: When you take big gaps between meals, you end up eating more the next meal and that's why you tend to eat all kinds of junk at the wrong time.

He interrupted, telling me that junk food was all that was available at his end.

Me: Can you not carry fruits or a packet of chana, singdana, makahana?

Rushabh: Per woh thodi khana hai, who to chakana hai (That's not food, it is something to be eaten along with alcohol).

Thus, I got to know that he consumed alcohol too, which he had not mentioned in the questionnaire.

Me: Eat food not just to fill your stomach, but also to give nutrition to your body. When you eat a fruit or chana versus a samosa, your body gets its dose of required nutrition.

By now, his body language had changed, and he went into listening mode.

Me: Fifth, your dinner time is sinfully late. What time does dinner get ready at your place?

Rushabh: Around 8:00 p.m.

Me: What time do you reach home?

Rushabh: Generally around 8:00 p.m.

Me: Then what stops you from having dinner immediately?

Rushabh: Abhi 8 baje to nastha karta hoo, to bhook kase lagegi. (I have snacks as soon as I get back home so I am not hungry.)

Me: Can you not skip your snacks and have dinner instead?

Rushabh: Itna jaldi khana!! phir baadme kya khaoo (If I have dinner so early, what will I eat if I feel hungry again).

Me: You will feel hungry, if you do not eat the right foods for dinner or if you don't sleep on time.

Rushabh: To kya abhi dinner bhi jaldi karna padega? (Do I need to have dinner early?)

Me: The right time to have dinner is by sunset. I am not asking you to have it at that time but suggesting you have it at least by 8:00 p.m.

He grinned.

Me: Sixth, why do you sleep so late?

Rushabh: Muzhe jaldi neend nahi atii, kya karu (I can't sleep early, what can I do).

I was waiting to answer this.

Me: It is due to your late and heavy dinner that your body is not ready to relax and sleep. Add to it the bright light emitted by your smartphone, which doesn't allow your eyes to relax and sleep.

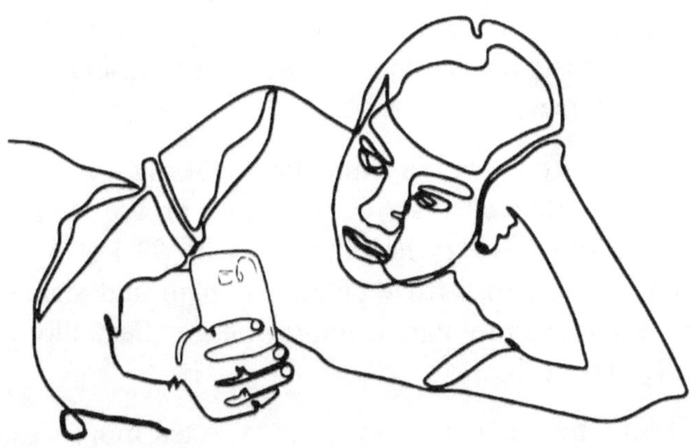

Rushabh: Per muzhe wohi time milta hai to connect with my friends (I only get time at night to connect with my friends).

This time I smiled, and I think he got the message, as he immediately said,

I can manage this, abhi weight loss karna hai to dost hi help karnege na (Who else can help me lose weight other than my friends).

Me: **Tathastu,**

He agreed to all that I had said, but then asked me the same question.

Rushabh: I will try doing all of this. Now, can you tell me how much time it will take for me to lose weight?

Me: Have patience and trust the process, you will eventually see the weight dropping.

I could sense that he was not completely convinced with my response, but he nodded in affirmation and this is how his fitness journey started.

He started with a bang by following everything diligently. He started seeing the results on the weighing scale. From 104 kgs, he came down to 99 kgs in two months. He also started gaining strength and stamina. His exercise form started improving, his flexibility got better day by day.

Still, he was not happy as he expected more weight loss and in the third month, he took a week's break to attend his cousin's marriage in Bengaluru and that break got extended from a week to a month to more than six months and all the good work that he had put in was lost within a flash.

The last I spoke to him, he said he was following an (ABC) diet, which helped him lose 10 kgs, but he gained more than that when he got back to his regular eating patterns. He was completely demotivated and gave up hope of ever being healthy!

When I look around, I see many people like Rushabh looking for quick results. There are many who start on a good note but do not continue for more than a month or two since they don't get the expected results (in a short period).

What needs to be understood is that fitness is never a temporary quick fix, but a continual process of ups and downs till you reach your goal. You must be consistent even after you achieve your goal.

To sum it up, the current scenario looks like this:

- **Sedentary** lifestyle

- **Low priority** towards health and fitness

- **Focusing** on **weight loss**

- Expecting **quick results** and open to **crash/fad dieting**

- **Inconsistent** and **short-term efforts**

- **Time constraints** and lack of the right resources

- **Low awareness** about nutrition

As we progress, we will elaborate on these points.

The next chapter is about "**Breaking the barriers**" and we will start with Rajesh's inspiring story and the way he overcame obstacles to achieve fantastic results.

Chapter 2

Break The Barriers

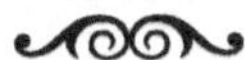

Barriers exist in your mind, train it right and your body will follow.

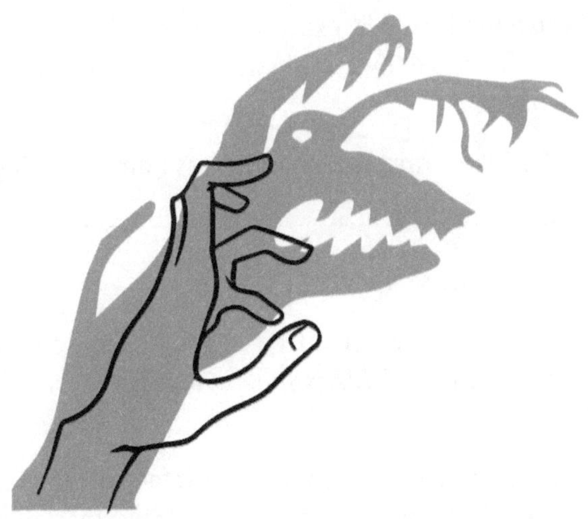

Let me tell you another story about Rajesh, a 50-year-old chartered accountant from Mumbai.

Rajeshji as we called him had always led a sedentary lifestyle and his work was the main reason behind it. Being glued to a desk and working continuously on accounting books had made him put on a lot of weight over the years. That lead to a few health issues and that was when he connected with us to lose a few kgs and lead a healthy life.

We did the body composition check and was surprised to see the numbers. It was not only about weight, which was almost 25 kgs more than ideal, his fat percentage was also on the higher side.

Rajesh: "I want to get fit, but I don't want to make drastic changes. I want to do it the right way and at a comfortable pace."

We decided on his exercise and meal plan and he registered for the 6:00 a.m. sessions, as that was the only time he had.

Rajesh: I will not miss a session unless I am travelling.

His journey started the very next day.

I still remember his first session; he was down in flat 10 minutes. (*This is how it usually is for all new participants*).

The way our sessions are conducted, there is a five to seven-minute warm-up, followed by five minutes of light to moderate cardio, followed by 30 minutes of strength training, and a cool-down session of another five to seven minutes. And we do four to five sessions a week spread across multiple batches. For the first week, we include only the warm-up, a bit of cardio, and cool-down, unless the participant is used to regular workouts.

As he started, he had his share of post-workout pain and soreness which all participants go through, but he did not make it an excuse to not attend sessions. Gradually, he started building stamina and in three weeks he could do the entire 45-minute workout.

This was well complemented by a balanced meal, which we had suggested with a focus on portion control and meal timing. His last meal was at 7:00 p.m. (Earlier, he used to have tea and biscuits.) He started seeing results and that gave him the confidence to focus better. Over a period, his strength and stamina had improved tremendously, that he could do the deadliest of strength training circuits just like a 25-year-old.

With these efforts, there were amazing results and he lost almost 23 kgs of body fat. (*Check his pictures and it will show you what he managed to achieve.*)

But this did not happen overnight!

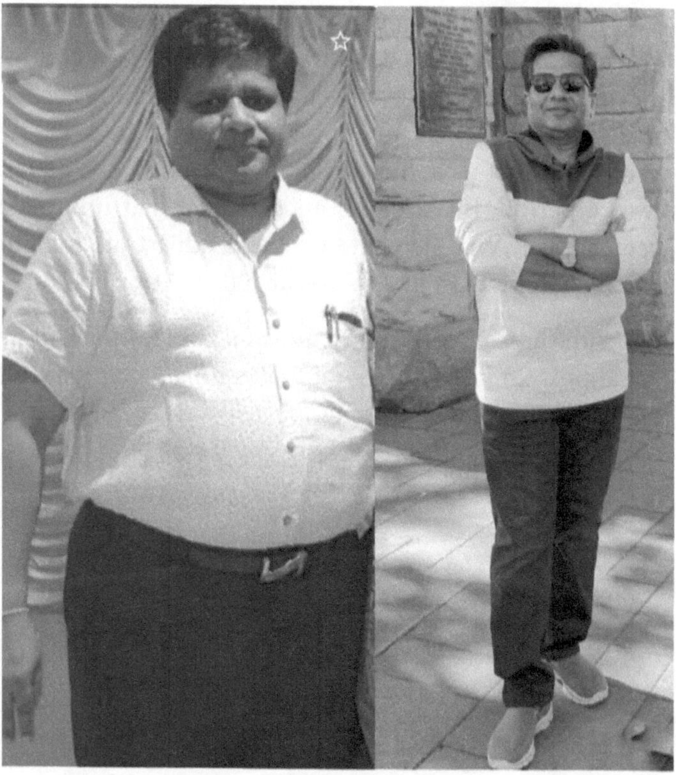

Transformation Story: Rajesh

It took more than nine months to get these results and he enjoyed every bit of the journey. More than the numbers, he adopted an active lifestyle which he follows even today.

I have seen many people who stop working out once their goal has been met, and then they gain back or put on more weight.

But this was not the case with Rajeshji. Even today, he is a regular for our 6:00 a.m. sessions. He follows his meal plans unless he is on vacation and that is why he has maintained his fitness levels, something which most people find tough to do.

"I have to change my wardrobe, as my old clothes are no longer fitting me," he told me one day, and I could sense his happiness.

When you look at overall fitness, you do not just lose weight or fat, but you lose inches too.

His digestion improved over time, so did his flexibility and sleep quality.

Few things to note about fitness, from this story:

- We all are busy but **we need to make time.** If we decide to, we will find the time.

- It is a process and you will go **through ups and downs** before you start seeing results.

- **It is not a onetime activity**, but a continual process, you need to be consistent, *and the results will follow you.*

- **It's never too late to start.** Rajesh started at the age of 50, and today he has the energy of a 25-year-old.

- And the last and the most important point, you must **start today** and not wait for Monday!

If this story inspired you to get started, let us get you started.

First, let's deal with common barriers:

Common Barriers: Time

"Will I gain more weight after I stop exercising?" is the most common question.

"But why do you want to stop exercising?" is my counter-question.

As I will not have the time to do it regularly!

If you are so busy that you cannot find 30 minutes for yourself, then what is the point of being so busy? Is it worth it? Think about it.

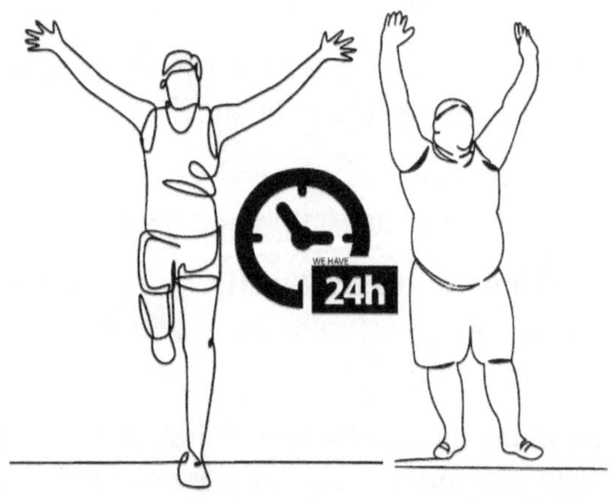

If Rajesh, a busy professional could make the time, I believe anyone can do that, at least give it a try. Rajesh always tells me one thing, *had I started this before.* ☺

Time will always be a concern, if and only if we do not plan it. We need just 30 minutes for a minimum of four days a week for exercise.

- That is just two hours per week.

- Eight hours a month, which is just one per cent of the total hours in a month.

Now tell me, is that **NOT POSSIBLE?**

Studies have said that on average we spend two hours a day on Social Media. This time *(where we investigate the lives of other people)* can definitely be used for our fitness.

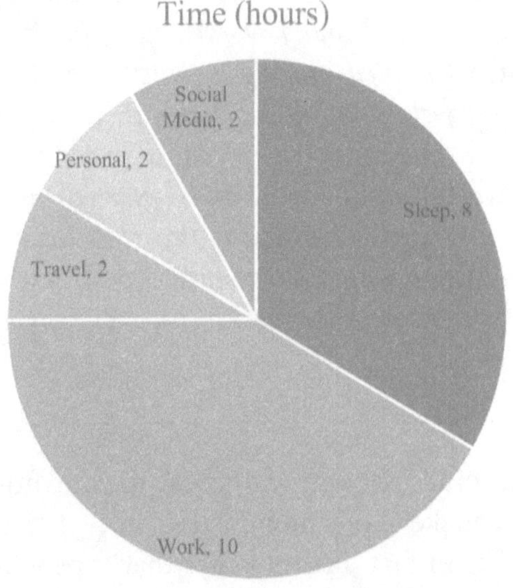

Still, there will be few who say, *"Time nahi hai" (I don't have time)*. I want to tell them one last thing:

Find 30 minutes now if you do not want to spend 30 days in a hospital later. It may look like an exaggeration, but I have seen people suffering from lifestyle diseases. And when the health report comes, even the busiest of people find time for a morning walk!

Regular exercise helps in building immunity and a strong musculoskeletal system over and above your weight loss goals.

Common Barriers: Money

There is never an end to our expenses.

When I started working 15 years back, earning 10k a month was my goal and I worked hard for it. I was so happy when I started making it, it felt like all the effort had paid off well. With added income, my expenses also grew, then a time came when I felt the need to make 15. Again, I worked hard for it, and I started making 15k. My expenses grew further and so the need to earn more. I realised that this was a never-ending cycle and I believe the same is the case with most of us, money is just never enough.

So, if you think that you will invest in your fitness only when you make more money, trust me, that time will never come. In fact, fitness is not that expensive, if you compare it to the benefits it offers.

Let's take an example of our very own Pedro and Fedro.

Pedro and Fedro work in a business firm and make around 30k a month and both have similar family commitments.

Pedro likes to stay fit, exercises regularly, and eats nutritious food. His fitness membership cost him 2k a month and his healthy eating grocery bills amounts to 4k a month, so he spends roughly 6k on his fitness. His regular fitness routine keeps him fit.

Fedro feels he does not earn much to invest in fitness, hence doesn't care to exercise and eat right. In fact, he tells Pedro not to spend on fitness and save that money to buy a car or go on vacation. Two years later, Fedro buys a new car.

If you had not wasted on a gym membership, aaj tumhari bhi gaddi hoti, (you too would have bought a car) he mocked Pedro.

A new car further added to his sedentary lifestyle and he reached the three-figure mark on the weighing scale in no time. One day, as he was getting out of his car in the office parking lot, he suffered a severe cramp in his lower back. It was so bad that he had to be escorted to the hospital using a stretcher (not even a wheelchair).

As per his diagnosis, he had developed a disc bulge. A major reason for this was his heavy weight and bad posture that put unwanted pressure on his spine. He went through immense pain for the initial two days. He had a lot of discomfort and could hardly sleep. After spending four days in the hospital, he was discharged and had to be on bed rest for another three days. After a week, he was able to walk on his own. A week later, he had an appointment with his doctor to discuss the next steps. His doctor showed him all his test reports which had been conducted when he was in the hospital.

Doctor: Fedro, your blood sugar levels and cholesterol are skyrocketing, and you are 30 kgs heavier than your ideal weight.

Fedro: I will do whatever you say to get well.

Doctor: You just need to lose weight.

Fedro: How?

Doctor: Here is the number of our dietician, go and visit her.

Fedro managed to get an appointment for the following week.

She looked at his reports, asked him a few questions, suggested a meal plan, asked him to start exercising and shared the contact details of a fitness trainer.

Fedro contacted the trainer and he put him on a special weight loss programme. Fedro finally started exercising and his meals were as per the plan: Clean and Balanced. Gradually, he started building his fitness and in six to nine months, he was able to strengthen his back and minimise (not eliminate) his back pain. Now he lives a healthy life, where he works out at least four days a week and eats a balanced meal.

Now let us look at the expenses he incurred during the whole six-month process:

He had spent almost Rs 1 lac to improve his health. Add to it the indirect expenses like office leaves, LOPs, etc, the overall cost was beyond Rs 1.25 lac in just six months. He was not able to pay the EMIs and had to literally sell off his car.

Had he taken care of his health like Pedro, he would have saved this money, plus avoided the pain which he had gone through.

Now let us compare this with Pedro's yearly expenses for fitness:

With Rs 6,000 a month, he spent just Rs 72,000 yearly, lesser than what Fedro had to shell out in six months. Add to it the amazing fitness levels he achieved, and the health benefits perceived.

If you look at this story, two things are evident:

1. You will have to take care of your fitness, **if not today then later** for sure. *(It's easier when you do it earlier)*

2. **Investing in fitness now** will help you minimise medical bills and the associated pain in future.

So accordingly make your choice.

Still, some may say, they do not have money. So, let me tell you, you can still take care of your fitness by going for a run or doing simple workouts in the garden or playground at no cost at all *(Check our Facebook page and you will find several exercise sequences which can be done by anyone)*. We have a chapter dedicated to exercise and you will find the required details.

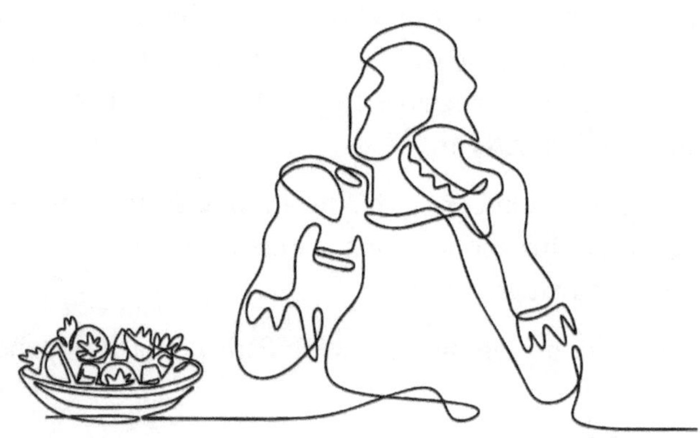

Eating healthy foods like fruits, vegetables, eggs and nuts will not cost you a bomb and can be managed with planning.

We have a chapter dedicated to nutrition and meals and it has the needed details.

Common Barriers: Lack of Interest

I get bored to lift weights, it is so monotonous. Is there any other way to get fit, asked Radha?

There are many, choose what interests you, I replied.

There are so many ways to exercise and it need not be restricted to the gym or a fitness centre. Many people do not find it interesting to lift weights, hence they shy away from gyms, which is fine.

As I said, there are different ways by which you can do it. It is not limited to:

- Running

- Cycling

- Playing a sport like football, cricket, hockey, tennis, badminton

- Swimming

- Dancing

- Brisk walking

- Karate/Krav Maga/Martial arts

- Boxing

- Hiking

- Wall climbing

- Yoga

- And even climbing trees.

There are more options. Choose what interests you and do it consistently and your body will thank you for the hustle. Besides, you will feel great doing something you like. It is like following your hobby.

You can always mix it up to avoid boredom. E.g.: Wall climbing + swimming can be one option, yoga + cycling, another.

One last thing:

Start slow (Don't get too excited and overdo on day 1.)

You may need to give the **initial push**, so do just that.

Once you start seeing changes in your body, your interest levels will go up and your fitness will run in **autopilot mode**.

Common Barriers: Lack of Motivation

Mere under se feeling ani chahiye, only then, I can do something, (I should get a feeling within, only then I can do something) said Sangeeta.

What she meant is she needed the motivation to get going.

Motivation means feeling good about doing a particular activity consistently without being reminded by anyone else.

It is also about having an **inner drive** to do something. This is possible only when you enjoy a particular activity.

There are a few techniques that can be used to stay motivated:

1. **Old is Gold:** It's time to test the quality of your high-end smartphone. Clean your house and

search for the old photo album and pick a photo that shows the best version of yourself.

(One tip: If you are in your forties, don't locate your school pics, that will be too much of an expectation, go back a maximum of 10 years.)

Now, use your camera and take the best possible shot of that photo and set it as your phone's wallpaper.

How does it help?

We see our mobile phone at least 100 times a day and when we do, we kind of see our best photo and slowly start believing that we can get back to that shape. This will push us to start.

This trick looks simple, but kind of motivates you to think positive and be optimistic about starting your journey. In fact, you can go one step further and make a photo collage as follows:

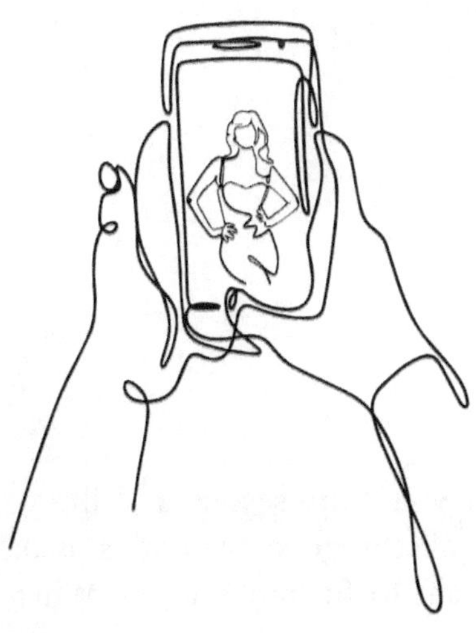

When you put this as your phone's wallpaper, it will definitely motivate you to take the effort to move from your current state to the desired state. You only need the stimuli to start and this collage will do that for you.

2. **Old clothes trial:** It's time to clean your wardrobe and locate your favourite old shirt or a pair of jeans which you loved wearing to college/office but can no longer wear it as you don't fit into it. Go back to the lovely memories you had wearing it. It may be a first date, or your best friend's wedding or a successful job interview. Next, wash it, iron it, and keep it in your cloth rack in such a way that every time you open the rack, it's visible.

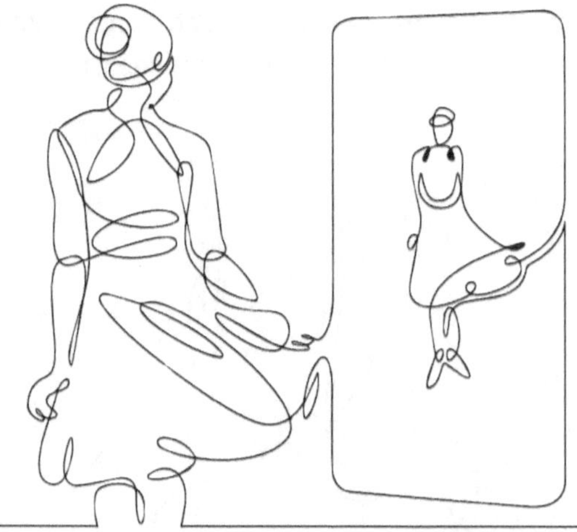

When you start seeing it daily, you will think about all the good memories associated with it and want to fit into it again. When this process happens daily for weeks together, there are high chances that the nostalgic feeling will push you to do something about your health and you may actually start exercising just to fit into those clothes.

Do consider any start as a good start.

3. Put things at stake:

One Sunday afternoon, you decided to take control of your health and immediately Googled a few good gyms in your locality. You shortlisted one and went there to check it out. You got impressed by the amazing facilities and decided to join it for three months. You went to the reception, filled the form, and took the three-month membership. You got home and told your family members about it. The chances are, they may have laughed, based on the many times in the past you had donated the yearly fees without even going for more than a week.

As the day progresses, you start casting doubts about whether you'd be able to do it.

This is the right moment to put things at stake.

Immediately get into a deal with your spouse, sibling, or your friend.

What's the Deal?

Tell them you have become serious about getting fit and will be regular at the gym.

To push yourself, you have kept thirty 500 rupee notes in a drawer and the day you miss the gym, they are free to pick one note.

You can decide whether it should be a 500 or a 2000 rupee note, depending on what will put the necessary pressure on you. For some, money may work, for others something else, identify what will challenge you and accordingly commit to it.

When you put things at stake, it motivates you to take action.

It's like Now or Never.

Also, it will make your family members understand your seriousness and they might support you in your journey. (*What else do you need, if you get home-cooked, nutritious food on a daily basis*).

4. Create Social pressure: Do you have a social media account?

Let's make the best use of it now. Generally, we are particular while posting on social media. Filters, spell checks, tags, etc, we check everything.

Once the post is done and we think it's a good one, we keep checking for likes and comments frequently. When someone posts a positive comment, we like it, whereas when anyone criticises us, we feel bad about it. Such is the impact of social media on our lives. This can provide the motivation to start our fitness journey.

How?

Put the following post on a Sunday morning *(or any day)*:

I have decided to get fit and plan to exercise every day for the next 90 days and will also put a post-workout pic. Wish me luck.

Social media is limitless and by putting this post up, you have committed to the world *(your friends, their friends)*. Now, this creates a good push to start exercising daily. Further, a good picture gets more likes, and this increases the motivation to do even better.

Also, since you have committed, you will find the best possible way to get the exercise done, as your friends *(some friends are special, you know what I mean)* keep a tab on you. You would not want anyone to laugh at you. This does create pressure and works in a good way. And the days you feel like giving up, suddenly you get this comment on one of your previous posts.

You are a source of motivation, seeing your pictures, I too feel like doing something for my health.

And your mood changes in a fraction of a second and you are all geared up to sweat it out again.

Does it really work?

I have a friend who had wanted to start a fitness centre for a long time. She had talked a lot about it but had not taken any concrete steps towards it. I happened to meet her over a coffee in Powai.

"What happened about your plan to start the fitness studio," I asked her.

"Oh ya, I want to start one, but somehow it's not working out," she replied.

"Are you so sure about it?"

"Definitely…"

"Can you announce this on your Facebook account?"

"What will happen if I do?

"Your studio will start for sure."

"Is it? Then let me post it right away."

She put up the following post:

I will have my fitness studio up and running at xxx location by xxx date.

Within the next eight months, I attended the opening ceremony of her studio.

How did this happen?

She quit procrastinating and started working on her plans. Since she had made the announcement, she also got support from a few of her friends in finding a place, getting a good interior designer, etc. So, it did not just keep her on her toes, but she also received the required support.

There is a famous dialogue from a Bollywood movie:

"Kehte hain agar kisi cheez ko dil se chaho ...to poori kainath use tumsee milane ke koshish mein lag jaati hai".

(It is said that if you want something from the heart...then the whole world takes effort to match it with you.)

The universe is ready to support you, you just make the announcement, start working on it and things will go your way. Such is the power of this tool.

5. **Kabhi khudko ainee me dekha hai? (Have you seen yourself in the mirror?)**

Do it now.

Stand in front of a full-size mirror and have a look at yourself for a good 10 minutes. You may even take longer if you are self-obsessed. Look at yourself from all angles, and then close your eyes standing there. Think about how you would want to look. Create a fit image of yourself.

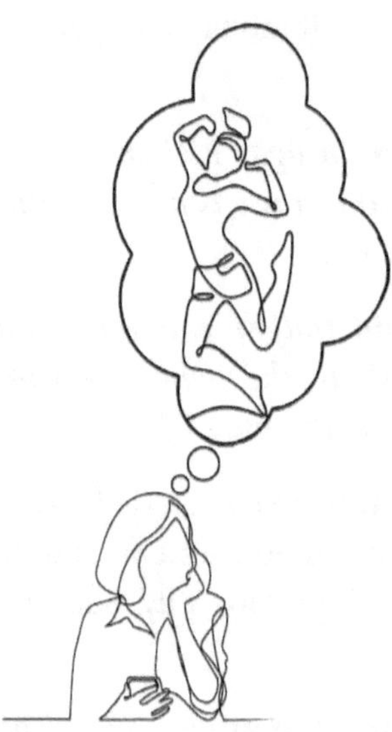

Open your eyes, take a blank paper and write down all the points you thought about:

For a few, it might just be about reducing the tummy.

A few might want to build strong arms

A few might want to reduce the flab on the arms, hips, etc.

A few might be pleased with the way they are.

Next, put today's date and a date by which you think you can become your fit self. Now, pin that paper to your washroom cabinet, just beside where you keep your toothbrush.

Every day, when you wake up and go to the washroom, you get to see that first, before checking your mail and messages.

So there are high chances you would go for a walk or a run after you finish your morning routine. You can also make copies of it and put it on your fridge, so the next time you plan to eat a scoop of ice cream or a piece of chocolate in the fridge, you get a view of that note first and that may stop you from eating junk.

If it has worked for you in terms of you being regular to the gym and focusing on avoiding junk, then you no longer need to continue this, you have found your motivation.

6. Self-Reward therapy:

"You know, my husband didn't even notice that I have lost weight. I purposely went in front of him wearing my old dress," said Rubina to her friend, while sipping a can of soda.

Kya fayda yeh weightloss ka, jab mere friends notice hi nahi karte, said Amrita to her mom. Aaj se sab band. (What's the point of this fitness when no one notices the difference?)

If you are one of the countless people who crave motivation for your fitness-related achievements, then this section is for you.

Everyone likes a pat on the back for the good things they do, but if you depend on someone else, then it can cause demotivation just like Rubina and Amrita.

This is where self-reward therapy comes in handy. It means rewarding yourself for the small success you achieve in your fitness journey.

And there is no better time to get one when you are ready to step out of your comfort zone, challenging yourself to improve your health.

If you train your mind to embark on this journey, setting small goals, and rewarding yourself for the smaller achievements, rather than waiting for the ultimate goal, you've already won the battle in your mind, and implementing it just becomes easier.

Further, rewards stimulate a feeling of achievement and it also motivates you to work much harder. Even the smallest of rewards can work wonders as you travel from milestone to milestone.

How do you do it?

- Set goals and allocate rewards for achieving each goal. You may want to break your main goal into smaller goals to make it manageable. (Goal setting will be covered in chapter six.)

- Make the reward meaningful to you. As a reward, a new pair of jeans may not hold as much motivation as a simple candlelight dinner in your favourite restaurant.

- Several small rewards, used for meeting interim goals, are more effective than relying solely on the bigger rewards that require more work and more time.

- Plan to celebrate, figure out how you'd cherish reaching your fitness goal. You may want to involve other people, tell them about it. The key is to anticipate your celebration and then keep it within sight all the time.

- Be honest with yourself. Reward yourself only if the milestone is achieved. Remember to keep your focus on building a habit, not just figuring out how to get the reward.

You will no longer need to depend on someone else to stay motivated.

I have covered the most common barriers and probable solutions to them. Now, the key is to hop on to your fitness journey immediately and tackle the barriers as they come.

Once you start, you will observe the positive changes to your body which will make you feel it's worth the effort. At this point, you may want to measure your progress and feel like standing on a weighing scale every now and then.

I am aware that the most common measures are fat loss/weight loss/inch loss. But do you know, fitness is much beyond these numbers!

How much weight you've lost or how quickly you lost it sounds interesting, but there is much more you need to look at when you talk about long-term fitness.

Don't worry, our next chapter is dedicated to telling you more about it.

Chapter 3
Think Beyond Scale

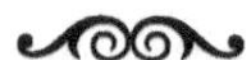

Let me tell you another story of a fitness freak, Jimmy.

Jimmy is a 30-year-old engineering graduate, working in a manufacturing firm. Apart from his work, he likes two things: Exercise and Food. He has been taking gym membership for almost three years now and his smartphone has all the food delivery apps. You name it and he has it. His social media has mainly two types of posts: His visit to yet another restaurant and a post-workout selfie with his workout buddy.

His fitness mantra is *"Khane ka aur gym me burn karneka"* *(Eat and burn calories in the gym)*

He spends almost 90 minutes at the gym each morning and has built a good physique over the years, something which he is proud of. His weight is also in the ideal range and his waistline is in control. By now, you may have got the impression that Jimmy is a fit guy.

Now read further.

He faces a lot of acidity and constipation issues which have impacted his sleep. But that does not stop him from hitting the gym. He does not feel fresh the entire day and feels tired, especially in the evening, and caffeine comes to his rescue. He is aware that it is due to his eating habits and one day he will work on it.

Re-evaluate your impression of Jimmy's fitness. What do you think about his overall health now?

Let me give my views:

- Jimmy has a good physique to flaunt and he looks strong, but what is the use of such fitness when his digestion has gone for a toss and he cannot sleep?

- Acidity can upset your day and constipation can ruin your mornings.

- For me, this is not real fitness, but just a visual appearance that creates a perception of being fit.

There are so many others like Jimmy who focus only on weighing scale-based results and take efforts accordingly. I am not saying one should not stand on a scale but look at other factors too. Fitness or holistic fitness is much beyond weight loss and this chapter talks about it.

Sasha: I've finally lost 10 kgs. I had told you this was a magical diet and see how it has worked wonders for me in just two months.

Me: That is great Sasha, tell me what you had for dinner yesterday.

Sasha: I have been skipping dinner ever since the day I started this diet. I only drink black coffee before bed.

Me: But skipping dinner is not a good idea.

Sasha: But this has helped me, look at my picture today.

Me: But you look so pale and you have got dark circles too.

Sasha: Oh, that's ok, kuch to khona padega na, kuch pane ke liye. (You will have to give up something to lose weight.) For me, losing the extra weight was a priority, now I will take care of other things.

I asked her one last question. Sasha, tell me, do you feel energetic at the end of the day?

She did not say a word and I got my answer.

This is how people are so desperate to look good on the weighing scale and thus they ignore other important aspects that include:

- How **energetic** do you feel in the afternoon and especially in the evenings? *(Most people tend to feel tired post 5:00 p.m. so they must have a cup of tea/coffee)*

- How **fresh do** you feel when you wake up? *(If you get sound sleep, your mornings will be blissful, or you always need a shot of caffeine)*

- How much **time** do you spend in the **washroom?** *(Constipation has become a common problem, most people don't have a bowel movement for days)*

- Do you get **sweet cravings** after your lunch/ dinner? *(Do you always reach out for a piece of chocolate/cookies post-lunch?)*

- Do you feel **acidic or bloated** once you wake up? *Or is it like goli ke bina (without acidity tablet), you don't start your day?*

- Do you keep **craving foods** throughout the day? *(You don't get satisfaction from your meals and you keep searching kitchen cabinets for something to snack on.)*

- Do you feel like **doing exercises**? *(Do you feel like being active or sitting in one place always?)*

- Do you experience **stiffness** in your neck and back regularly?

- Do you feel **breathlessness** on and off?

- Are you able to **sleep peacefully** at night or you play the role of nightwatchman? *(Do you consume sleeping pills?)*

- How good is your **mood?** *(How do you behave with your family? Are you like Ram at the office and Ravan at home?)*

- How good is your **posture**? *(Can you sit without back support? Can you stand without leaning on a wall?)*

- Do you **get tired** of doing daily activities? *(You might lift heavy weights in the gym, but if you cannot climb four steps with a grocery bag in hand, then what is the point?)*

- How good is your **flexibility**? *(Are you able to reach under the table to pick up a fallen object or do you need help?)*

- How good is your **immunity?** (*Do you sneeze due to slight weather changes?*)

- How good is your **stamina?** (*You can run on a treadmill for 30 minutes, but you pant on climbing a few steps.*)

- Do you **breathe right** using full lung capacity? (Is one nostril blocked and you breathe only through the other?)

- Do you feel **lethargic** and always stay in bed or do you feel strong and fresh?

- How good is your **digestion**? Do you feel uneasy or sleepy after meals?

- How regular and comfortable is your **monthly cycle?**

- Are you **ageing gracefully**? (*Do you look and feel like you are in your forties when you are in your thirties?*)

- Are you able to **focus on your work** or do you get distracted thinking of your weight?

- How do you **manage stress?** Can you handle stress well or do you crumble?

Take time to go through this, and if you don't score a brownie point in at least 80 per cent of the above items, then your *Dole-Shole* is of no use.

Most tend to overlook these important parameters and only run behind weight loss. One may get instant gratification when he/she sees a drop in weight like Sasha, but if any of the above-mentioned parameters are not right, then you will not enjoy life.

Imagine taking pills every day for acidity. I know a few who carry acidity pills and take them post-lunch every day.

When asked, why don't you reduce the oil and masala from your food?

"Masala nahi to kya maja, ye goli hai na, pura acidity nikal deta hai one min me".

(There is no fun in eating if there is no spice. Taking an acidity tablet gives instant relief).

Your energy levels depend on what you've eaten the entire day rather than your 50 kg bench press. The right food gives you good energy, so if you eat five to six portions of balanced meals, your health will be good. We will talk more about meals in a separate chapter.

Do it the right way:

- **Sleep** is one of the major influencers and an often overlooked parameter of fitness. Ensure that you get seven to eight hours of sound sleep every single day. One way to get this done is to have dinner three hours before you hit the bed. Stay away from gadgets at least an hour before you sleep. *(One chapter is dedicated to sleep.)*

- **Good digestion** impacts several things including your mood and daily routine. Many feel constipated and bloated for weeks and one reason is the time at which they have their meals. A good digestive system ensures the efficient absorption of nutrients in your body. *(Will talk more about it in the upcoming chapters.)*

- **Flexibility** is often an overlooked factor; in fact, it is always compromised in favour of strength. If you can do 20 push-ups but are not able to touch your toes, then it's not complete fitness.

  If you do not work on your flexibility, there are chances that you'd experience muscle sprains and are more prone to injury. Adding warm-up and stretching sequences to your exercise routine will help in improving your flexibility. Also, maintain correct posture and don't be sedentary.

- Over and above your physical fitness, your peace of mind, or what we call **stress levels** need to be in control. If you do not get bothered by unwarranted expectations regarding weight loss, it can help you destress.

  I have seen people get depressed about not losing weight. Practising deep breathing techniques and mediation as part of your morning routine and setting reasonable expectations can help manage stress.

This list can go on, but if you look at the above points, you will realise that nowhere are we talking about exercise *(other than warm-up and stretching)*.

Our overall fitness is way beyond physical fitness and exercise. Hence, when you set a fitness goal, think beyond weight loss, and focus on these non-scale parameters. And if anyone tells you that they *have a magical diet that will help you lose X kgs in one month*, ask them whether it will help you improve these non-scale parameters.

And if they tell you, kya farak padta, weight loss to ho jayega? (How does it matter, you will lose weight anyway?)…feel free to share your knowledge on the same, the way I did ☺.

Chapter 4

How to Start

I have conquered all my obstacles and am ready to embrace an active lifestyle. Tell me how I can start, asked Ketaki, as she was about to get into an elevator to the office.

Ketaki, an HR professional, is an old friend and now a coach with Fitnessmessengers. Let me tell you her inspiring journey as narrated by her.

Ketaki: I am breaking down my journey into a few stages:

Stage 1: Before Marriage

Sports, exercise, and dance were a part of my routine. I was very conscious of what I ate and how I looked at that stage of life. The only things I had to manage were my job, workouts, meals, and weekends. And since I was working out regularly and taking care of my meals, I was very much on my ideal fitness parameters.

Weight: 55 Kgs

Stage 2: Post-Marriage

New life, new family, new customs, new culture, I was slowly adapting to it; initially, I was conscious about my workouts and meals. However, as days passed, I started getting careless about my meal timings and regular exercise, the primary reason being laziness. And the family events and outing in the first year added to my excuses.

Weight increased from 55Kgs – 58Kgs, body fat up by almost 4%

Stage 3: Maternity

It was time to feel happy and I was on top of the world. And as happiness comes with a celebration, so was mine but it was an extended one ☺. Further, eating became a ritual under the pretext of food cravings. Add to it the lack of exercise and my weight increased further.

Weight increased from 58kgs to 85kgs (27Kgs)

Stage 4: Post Maternity

I was gifted with a beautiful healthy daughter. Like all moms, my life completely changed after that. I was enjoying that phase of my life, but in the process, I completely ignored my health and when I think about it, I find that the same is the case with almost all new moms today.

Almost a year passed by and I realised that my fitness levels had gone for a toss. I used to breathe heavily when I spoke to anyone at a stretch. I was not able to carry my baby for a long time due to backache. It was so bad that I could not even climb one floor up to get home. I was completely demotivated, and the post-maternity hormonal changes added to it. Life was getting tough and then one fine day I decided that enough is enough, I need to work on my fitness.

I started eating home-cooked food, stayed away from tea and beverages, exercised three to four days a week, and most importantly, had dinner before 8:00 p.m. Doing this helped me lose the maternity weight. I reduced from 85 to 72 kgs in one year. But then, I became overconfident, which happens with most people. Since I had lost good weight, I started celebrating, became casual about my workouts, the simple reason being, I believed that even if my weight did increase, I could reduce the same way... but that never happened. Thankfully, I did not gain more weight but was stuck at 72 kgs, which was almost 15kgs more than my ideal weight.

Stage 5: Four years after maternity

My work schedule and my little one kept me busy for the entire day. Working mothers with no domestic help will understand what I am talking about. It was challenging to have my regular meals on time and most of my meals were from the cafeteria which had low nutrition value and high calories.

I started feeling lethargic and demotivated. Stagnancy and low motivation had overshadowed me. I wanted to lose weight desperately and in that rigour, I would always start my weight loss regime in full swing but that would fade off in two weeks due to some or reason or the other: Family, work, etc. I also tried all kinds of diets but that did no good for me. Whenever I did those diets, I'd lose two to three kgs but I would get back to square one within a few days. This further frustrated me, and I completely gave up on my fitness.

That was when I came across Fitnessmessengers and started interacting with Bhushan. He spoke about how critical it was for me to do something about my fitness now. He showed me a few examples of his clients who had gone through a transformation after maternity. Seeing real-life examples inspired me and I told him that I also want to do it. He began by asking about my muscle and fat levels for which I had no answers. I said that I just wanted to lose belly weight. He explained that transformation was all about building lean muscle and losing fat. Your weight can be either muscle weight or fat weight, hence you shouldn't just focus on weight but look at building muscle and losing fat. This statement changed my perspective and shifted my focus from weight loss to healthy weight loss. I was still not sure whether it would work and thought of giving it a try and that's how my transformation process started.

I was given a meal plan which had five to six smaller portions a day and the main factor was to have my last solid meal by 7:30 p.m. (versus the 9.30–10 pm as I usually did). From my initial two to three meals, I was having almost six meals a day. Initially, I was surprised, as I felt I had to eat so much and I would gain more weight, rather than lose it. I also started doing the functional training workouts and within 20 days, I started seeing some results. Gradually the intensity of my workouts increased and so did my adherence to the meal plans and within six months, I lost almost 15 kgs of fat and added 7% lean muscle mass to my body.

I had achieved my goal; I was back at 55kgs and even till today I have managed to maintain that weight by following an active lifestyle. It does go up and down by a kg or more, but that's how it works.

My message to all those who are looking to get fit:

START TODAY, TAKE THE FIRST STEP, TRUST THE PROCESS, BE CONSISTENT AND YOU WILL SEE AMAZING RESULTS.

Thanks.

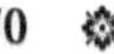

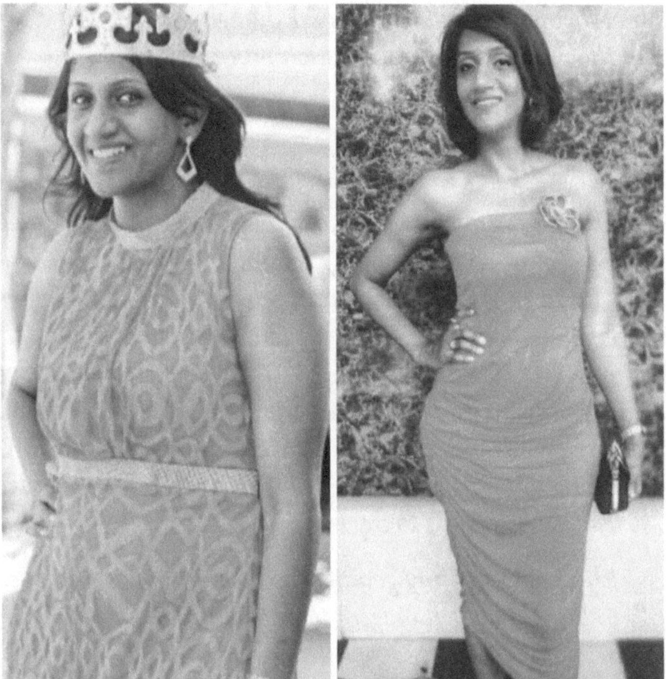

Transformation Story: Ketaki

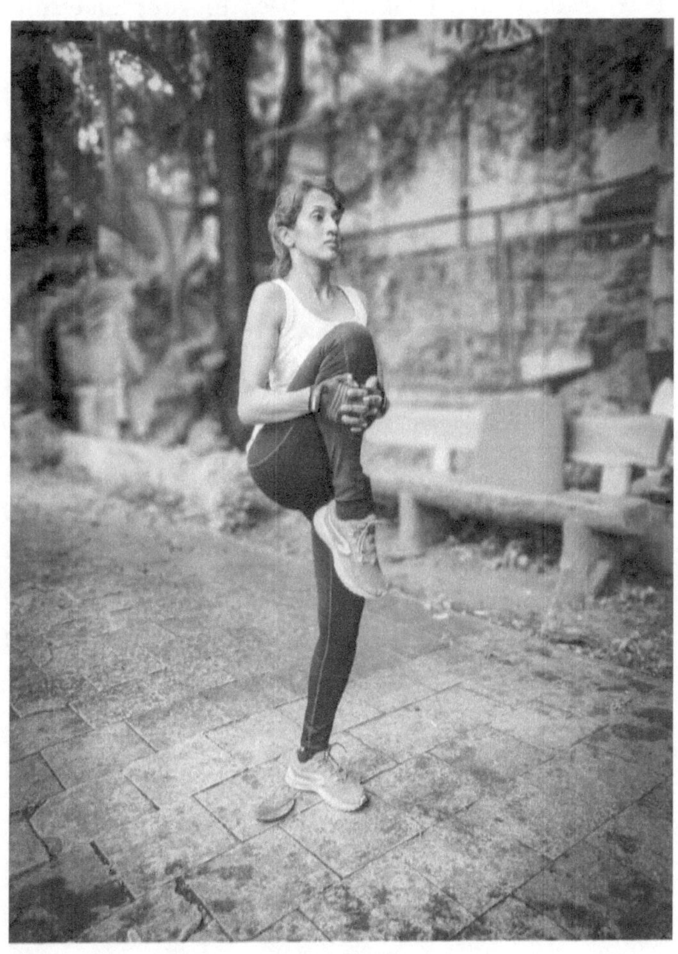

Coach Ketaki

- Isn't her story **motivating?**

- How many of you can **relate to her?**

- Moms, did it take you back to **your maternity days?**

- Did it remind you about the frustration of **frequent weight gain and weight loss cycles** despite following strict diets?

- And finally, did it not give you hope that **You too can do it?**

So, **let's do it.**

By now you would have identified the barriers and I am sure would have found ways to deal with them.

If you are still not there, go back to the previous chapter, read it again, implement the suggestions and you will be in the right frame of mind to start your journey.

As we move ahead, there are a series of chapters that will take you through the entire process.

Read a chapter, take learnings from it, start implementing the lessons, then move to the next one.

Chapter 5

Self-Assessment

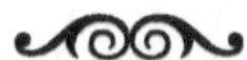

Let me tell you about Saurav, a software engineer working in a multinational company. He loves to play badminton on weekends and as such looks fit. We were discussing fitness in general on a Saturday morning.

Saurav: I am very fit, I just checked my weight and it's in the normal range.

Me: That's great, but what is your fat percentage.

Saurav: It will also be in the normal range! abhi weight thik hai, to sab thik hi hona hai na!

(As my weight is in the normal range, other parameters will also be fine.)

Me: Not necessarily.

Saurav: Impossible!

Me: Let's check it right away

(I removed the muscle and fat scanner from the drawer.)

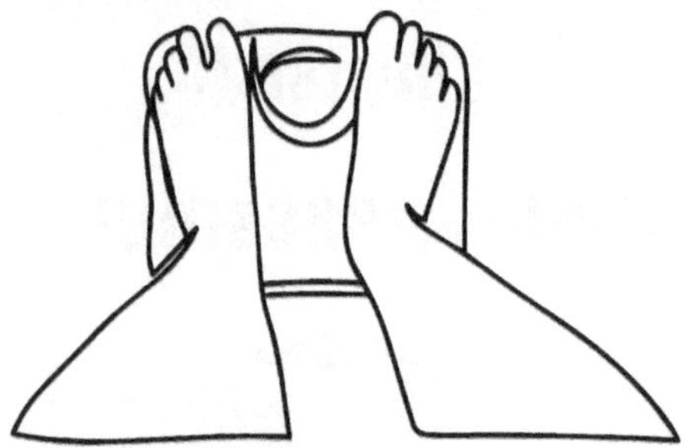

Saurav: What is this now?

Me: This is a magical machine and will tell you many things about your body.

He was reluctant to check it, but just because I reminded him about a higher fat percentage, he got ready to check. He must have thought, "Abhi dikhata hu isko." (I will prove him wrong.)

He stood on the scanner and I took the readings.

Saurav: See, I told you all is fine.

I showed him the readings:

- Weight – 76.4 kgs

- Total body fat – 28.2%

- Subcutaneous fat – 20.6%

- Visceral fat – 12%

- Muscle – 30%

- BMI – 26.9

- Body Age – 46

- Resting Metabolic rate (RM) – 1701

Saurav: I do not know what these numbers mean.

Me: Do not worry, let me explain.

Let's start with **weight,**

To understand whether you are at your ideal weight, there is a simple calculation.

Ideal weight:

- For females: height in cms – 105

- For males: height in cms – 100

Me: Saurav, since your height is 170 cm your ideal weight is 70 kgs, which means you are overweight by 6 kgs. Like I said, weight is not the only parameter of fitness, as weight can go up even when muscle mass goes up, which is in fact healthy. Whereas, when you lose muscle which is not healthy, it can result in weight loss too.

Saurav: So, what more should we look at?

Me: Let's focus on other parameters too.

Total Body Fat is the overall fat in your body. The ideal range for females is 25%, while for males it is 15%. It differs according to age, but I have quoted an average which is a good enough start. While some fat is definitely required, excess causes damage. Saurav, in your case, the fat percentage is on the higher side, so your focus should be on reducing it.

There are further categorisations of fat.

Subcutaneous fat is the layer of fat just below your skin. The range should be less than 15%. It's higher in your case. Have you seen anyone with a double chin?

Saurav: Yes. (He rolled his hand over his chin.)

Me: This fat is one of the reasons.

Then there is **Visceral fat**. It is considered the riskiest of all fat and is the fat surrounding your vital organs. It is also called killer fat as the higher the presence of this fat, it puts more pressure on the organs.

A range of 2–4% is normal. Anything above this is dangerous and needs to be worked on. The functioning of the organs gets impacted over time and can lead to multiple issues.

Muscle is the strength of the body. For men, it should be at least 33% and for women, it should be at least 30%. Higher the muscle, better strength and stability, and less chance of fat occupying the body. Muscle occupies a lower volume than fat, hence you look toned when you have more muscle. There is scope for you to work on your muscle strength.

Body Mass Index (BMI) is the ratio of height and weight and an ideal range is 18.5–24.9.

Body age shows how quickly we are aging and should ideally match our actual age. A different number indicates that your health parameters need to be worked on.

Since your other parameters are not in the ideal range, your BMI and Body Age are not in the ideal range.

Resting Metabolism (RM) means the number of calories your body needs when it is at rest. Even when you are resting your body needs the energy to do regular activities like breathing, brain function, or even reading this book. A lower RM indicates that your body needs fewer calories and it also means that your weight loss journey will be slower.

Saurav: So many things to look at.

Me: Exactly, that is the human body. It's not so straightforward to assess your fitness just by looking at your weight. Hence, when you identify your fitness goal, all these parameters need to be considered.

Saurav: Thanks, this is an eyeopener. Can you also help me in setting my fitness goal?

Me: Sure…let us start right away.

Take a pen and paper, our next chapter is about setting fitness goals.

Chapter 6
Setting Fitness Goals

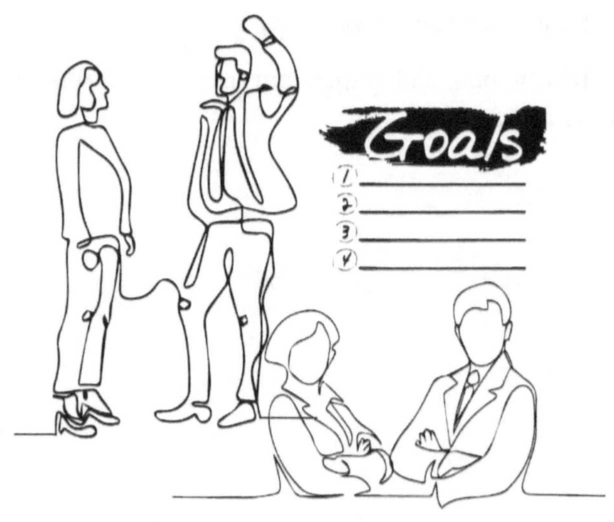

Tell me Saurav, what's your fitness goal?

Saurav: I just want to get fit.

Me: Now, this is a generic statement, what do you mean by *Get Fit*?

How will you measure your progress?

Saurav: You mean, I need to specify some numbers?

Me: You need to clearly define your fitness goal.

Saurav: We do it for our million-dollar projects, it's a complex process.

Me: But does it help?

Saurav: It does.

Me: Your body is priceless! Don't worry, I will make it simple for you. Goals help you stay focused, especially when things don't go as expected. Like we have our business goals, personal goals, academic goals, project goals, vacation goals, we can have fitness goals too.

I am sure you must have heard about this concept: Goals need to be SMART (*Specific, Measurable, Attainable, Realistic/Relevant and Time-Bound*).

Let's start the process and at the end, we will check whether they are SMART.

The first step is to do a self-assessment to understand where you currently stand in terms of fitness. It will give you the right starting point.

Me: As discussed, I will help you set your fitness goal, are you ready?

Saurav: Yes, I am eager to begin the process.

Me: Let's start with scale-based parameters:

Parameters	Current scenario	Ideal scenario	Change
Weight	76.4 kgs	70 kgs	Reduce 6 kgs
Body Fat	28.2%	15%	Reduce 13%
Subcutaneous Fat	20.6%	15%	Reduce 5%
Visceral Fat	12%	2–4%	Reduce 8%
Muscle	30%	33%	Gain 3%
BMI	26.9	18.5–24.9	Reduce by 2 points
Body Age	46	Your current age	

Let's descriptively set your goal:

Your fitness goal is to build 3% muscle mass and reduce 13% body fat in the next 6–9 months.

Saurav: Looks cool.

Me: Hold on, we are not done yet.

Saurav: What is missing now?

Me: Think beyond the scale too. (Non-scale parameters.)

Let me rephrase your fitness goal:

Your fitness goal is to build 3% muscle mass and reduce 13% body fat in the next 6–9 months. You should be able to experience strength and flexibility to aid your body movements while doing your daily tasks. You should drink three to four litres of water and get seven to eight hours of sound sleep. Your digestive system should be good enough that you should not experience bloating, acidity on a regular basis. Most importantly, you should feel good about your journey and not get stressed about losing weight.

Saurav: Now this looks like a complex project.

Me: Yes, but the only difference is, here you are the customer, unlike your software projects.

Now let's check the SMART principle:

Is it Specific?

-Gain 3% muscle mass and reduce 13% body fat are specifics with no ambiguities. Also, the non-scale parameters are listed objectively.

Is it Measurable?

-Fat and muscle improvements can be measured using a machine, similarly, water and sleep can be measure in litres and hours respectively. The same is the case with frequencies/instances of acidity and bloating.

Is it Attainable?

-It looks attainable as a good time frame is considered. Also drinking three to four litres of water and sleeping seven to eight hours a day is possible with proper planning.

Is it Realistic?

-We are looking for real improvements in terms of muscle and fat and nowhere have we mentioned achieving six packs which would look unrealistic in this time frame.

Is it Time-bound?

-A time window of 6–9 months is mentioned, and the subsequent plan needs to be made accordingly.

Saurav: Thanks, so can I have a plan for the next 6–9 months?

Me: We are not yet done.

Saurav: What is pending?

Me: Planning for 6–9 months will not make sense; we need to break your bigger goal into multiple interim goals.

Saurav: You mean project milestones.

Me: That's right, let's define milestones for this million-dollar project.

Milestones are like pit stops to assess your progress; it also allows you to have smaller successes on the path towards your ultimate goal. Basically, it is about breaking your goals into smaller goals and achieving them one by one.

A car journey from Mumbai to Panchgani (a hill station in Maharashtra) is about five hours. For a few, driving at a stretch is fun, but for others like me, it can be a task. So, I generally take two breaks: One on the expressway for fuel and the other in Pune for a meal.

So, when I refuel my car, my first milestone is met, and when I have a meal at Way Down South, an amazing place in Pune, my second milestone is met, and finally, when I reach the land of strawberries, my ultimate goal is met.

These breaks or milestones as I call them allows me to have a comfortable journey. At the end of the first milestone, I can check whether I am on time and how much time I can afford to spend on the second break for meals, or should I skip it so that I reach my hotel by the check-in time.

I am sure, many people plan their vacations accordingly. So, extending the same logic to your fitness journey can make it comfortable, allowing you to plan/re-plan your next steps.

Why are they important?

Your goal can take a good amount of time, like 6–9 months in Saurav's case. It may make you think, *"abhi time bahot hai" (I have lots of time)* and this can delay the start. Also, you would need to check at regular intervals whether you are making steady progress as per the plan and if any corrections are needed.

In Saurav's case: The overall goal is to reduce fat by 13% and gain muscle by 3% in 6–9 months plus focus on achieving the non-scale parameters.

This can be broken into milestones:

First Milestone: End of 1st month – 0.5% muscle gain and 1.5% fat loss, consume 2 litres water and get 7 hours of sleep every day.

What it means is Saurav will work to add half a per cent muscle mass and lose around one and a half per cent fat. Also, he will drink 2 litres of water daily and get at least 7 hours of sleep.

You can again compare it to the SMART principle to be sure. When you set these smaller goals *(milestones)*, you can plan accordingly and conquer them. Do remember the self-reward system once you achieve it. Also, if you don't achieve a planned milestone, you can re-plan the activities for the next milestone and still manage to be on target for your ultimate goal. (*The way we manage our expenses on vacation, if we spend more on day 1, we try to spend less on the remaining days.*) IT professional working in agile-based projects will appreciate the value of milestones *(Sprints in their language)*.

Similarly, identify the next set of milestones.

Second Milestone: End of 2nd month – 1% muscle gain and 2.8% fat loss, 2.2-litres water, 7 hours sleep with bedtime before 11:00 p.m.

Third Milestone: End of 3rd month – 1.5% muscle gain and 4.5% fat loss, 2.5-litres water, 7 hours sleep with bedtime before 11:00 p.m. and dinner by 9:00 p.m.

Fourth Milestone: End of 4th month – 2% muscle gain and 5.5% fat loss, 3-litres water, 7.5 hours sleep with bedtime before 10:45 p.m. and dinner by 8:30 p.m.

Fifth Milestone: End of 5th month – 2.5% muscle gain and 7% fat loss, 3.25-litres water, 8 hours sleep with bedtime by 10:30 p.m. and dinner before 8:00 p.m.

Sixth Milestone: End of 6th month – 3% muscle gain and 8.5% fat loss, 3.5-litres water, 8 hours sleep with bedtime by 10:15 p.m. and dinner before 7:45 p.m.

Seventh Milestone: End of 7th month – 3.25% muscle gain and 9.5% fat loss, 3.75-litres water, 8 hours sleep with bedtime by 10:00 p.m. and dinner by 7:30 p.m.

Eight Milestone: End of 8th month – 3.5% muscle gain and 11.5 % fat loss, 4-litres water, 8-hour sleep with bedtime by 10:00 p.m. and dinner by 7:30 p.m.

Ninth Milestone: End of 9th month – 3.5% muscle gain and 13% fat loss, 4-litres water, 8-hour sleep with bedtime by 10:00 p.m. and dinner by 7:00 p.m.

(Add non-scale parameters too)

Saurav: I have something to achieve for each month.

Me: Absolutely, if things go right, you can always continue with your efforts, but if things go wrong, you get an opportunity to make the required corrections to your actions. Another benefit is it allows you to celebrate process victories which are essential for you to stay focused on your journey.

So, Goals – Milestones, What Next?

Break them further!

Break your milestones into interim milestones.

From **month level goal**, come to a **week level goal.**

E.g.: if the 1st milestone is: 0.5% muscle gain and 1.5% fat loss, 2 litres water and 7 hours sleep

The weekly targets can be:

First Interim Milestone: End of Week 1: 0.1% muscle gain and 0.25% fat loss, 1-litre water, and 6.5 hours sleep.

At the end of week 1, check how you are progressing. If it's going as per plan, then great and if not, re-plan.

Second Interim Milestone: End of Week 2: 0.1% muscle gain and 0.5% fat loss, 1.25-litre water, and 6.5 hours sleep. *(Not all parameters can change simultaneously.)*

Third Interim Milestone: End of Week 3: 0.3% muscle gain and 1% fat loss, 1.5-litres water, and 7 hours sleep.

Fourth Interim Milestone: End of Week 4: 0.5% muscle gain and 1.5% fat loss, 2-litres water, and 7.25 hours sleep.

Add non-scale parameters too.

So, Goals – Milestones – Interim Milestones, What Next?

Plan actions for each interim milestone and progress towards achieving them.

Taking action is what will help you achieve your goals; else they remain fantasies.

When you have targets on weekly basis, you can plan actions for 7 days, which is feasible compared to planning for 30 days or even 6–9 months.

Let us look at what actions we can plan for the first-week target: Week 1: 0.1% muscle gain and 0.25% fat loss, 1-litre water, and 6.5 hours sleep.

Actions:

Start exercising, either go for a run or join a gym.

1. Eat 5–6 portion-controlled meals.

2. Keep a water bottle handy and a reminder system, so you can drink water at regular intervals.

3. Finish your work early, so you can be in bed on time.

Do not make frequent changes to your lifestyle, else it will be difficult to follow them consistently.

E.g.: if you are used to sleeping at 1:00 a.m., plan to sleep by 12:30 a.m. or 12:15 a.m. in the first week and gradually sleep earlier week on week.

You can further break your actions into daily tasks and hourly tasks as required.

So, the cycle is **Goals – Milestones – Interim Milestones – Actions.**

Activity: Write down your fitness goals.

Goal Setting

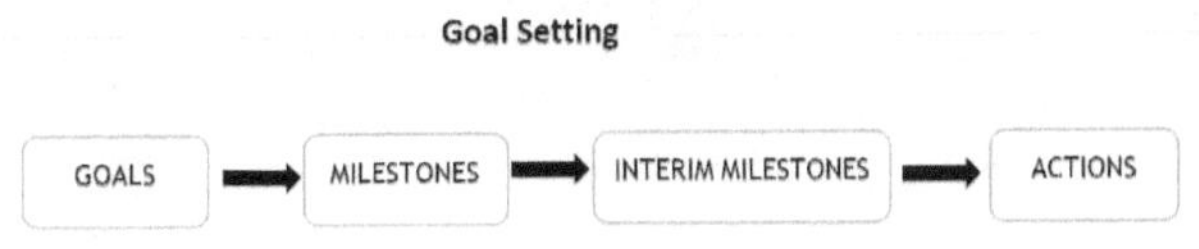

Stay tuned as we talk about an interesting topic in our next chapter: Exercise to get stronger.

Chapter 7
Exercise to Get Stronger

I want to look toned, mere muscles dikhna chaiyee, (My muscles should be visible) exclaimed Raj in Mumbai style.

Whereas somewhere in Lucknow, Anil said, "I should just look big, bicep ka size bada chaiyee." (My biceps should grow.)

Lilly, an old Goa resident was of the opinion: I do not want to look manly; I just want to have a flat tummy.

Areef from Noida was behind a six-pack: I want six-pack abs, baki kuch nahi chaiyee. (Nothing else matters.)

And Munro from the pink city felt he was overall fit, bas thoda pet kam karna hai. (I just need to tone my stomach.)

There is so much variety, isn't it?

Different people have different expectations about their fitness, but one aspect is common: EXERCISE.

Before we get there, let us talk about this term which has become common nowadays:

"Sitting is the new smoking."

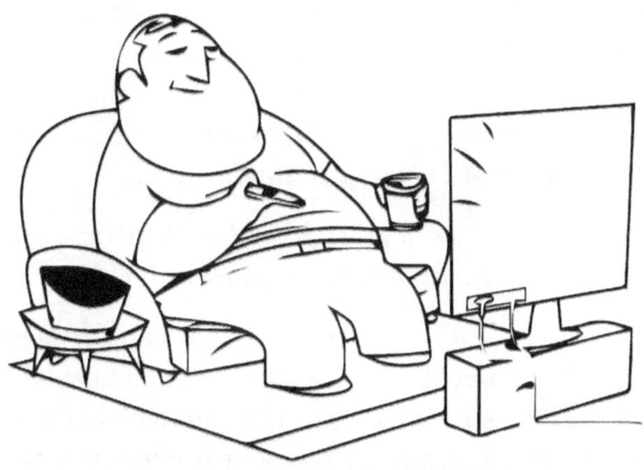

We are aware of the effects of smoking on our body, now it is time to know about the other part. Lifestyle diseases like diabetes, blood pressure, back pain, neck pain, heart ailments, and many others are attributed to lack of physical activity.

We have been hearing a lot about **LIFESTYLE DISEASES** nowadays, so what is it?

It's the way we live our life.

Can these diseases be avoided if we live the right way? **Of course.**

Doing 40 minutes of exercise at least four days a week, eating right, being active and not being sedentary have been found to be effective in preventing these diseases. Over and above, exercise helps you build muscle, improve posture, change your mood, manage your weight, and eventually, make you healthy.

I was talking to Partha, a banker by profession. He has been trying to lose weight for a while, but his lifestyle was in a bad state. Attribute it to his desk job, or his tendency to eat sweets, it was just not helping. He had come in for a fitness consulting session and I made him stand on the muscle and fat scanner.

Partha: Obesity to huamre khandan ki parampara hai (runs in our family)…it's in our genes.

Me: Have you not seen identical twins with the same set of genes but different physical activities and talents? Your genes do contribute to your health, but that's not the only factor. It also depends on how much effort you take to manage your fitness. Woh wala jeans ko utar ke fek do aur ye naya wala jeans le lo I replied in a funny way. (Replace the jeans with a new one.)

Partha: Okay, I get it, but tell me, which is the best exercise for me to get good results?

Me: The one which you will not miss (I replied in a filmy style).

Partha: You mean daily?

Me: At least four days a week.

Partha: Let us do it from Monday and the discussion continued.

Getting fit is no longer a choice, it's mandatory. And if you put in the right efforts, it is not impossible.

Exercise

There are different types of exercises, but for the simplicity of this discussion, I am dividing it into two parts: Cardio and Strength Training.

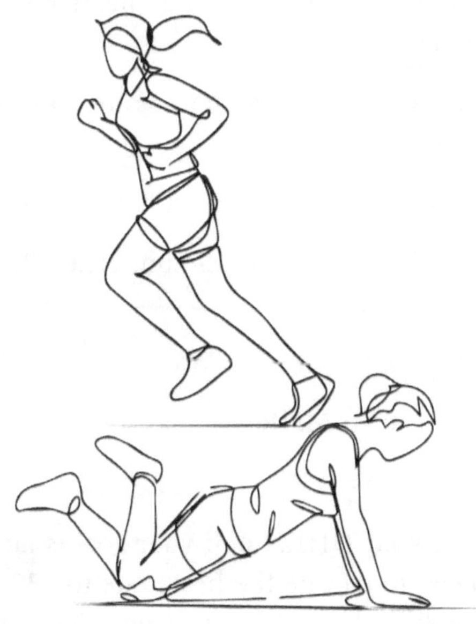

Cardio

When you say you run on a treadmill or you cycle, you are doing a cardio exercise.

Cardio or cardiovascular activities are a set of exercises that increases your heart rate. Running, cycling, brisk walking, playing recreational sports like badminton, cricket are examples of cardio exercises.

These exercises help you build stamina.

But do they help with fat loss?

Let's understand this concept:

While exercising, when your heart rate increases beyond a certain threshold called the optimum fat-burning zone, your body starts burning fat. Hence the intensity of your workout should be such that your heart rate is in the optimum zone.

Use this formula to calculate your optimum fat-burning zone:

220 – Your Age = Maximum Heart Rate (MHR)

And 70% of MHR is your Optimum Heart Rate (OHR) for a good fat burn.

E.g.: if your age is 35,

220–35 = 185 is your MHR

OHR = 70% of 185 = 130

So, 130 is your OHR. So, if your goal is fat-burning, then you need to elevate the heart rate to 130 beats per minute. Anything below that will not give you the fat-burning benefit. This also explains why walking is not the right exercise for fat loss, as during walking, the heart rate does not elevate much, so it does not aid fat loss.

Now you know why uncle Sam, despite walking for two hours in the garden every single day, still carries his paunch.

The easiest way to measure your heart rate: Set the stopwatch to a min and count your pulse.

You can also use fitness devices available at your end.

While doing cardio exercises, our body utilises a lot of oxygen, hence there is a good calorie burn. The more oxygen consumed, the more calories burnt. That is why you burn more calories after jogging. Oxygen intake is also proportional to the heat expenditure, hence you sweat when you jog.

Cardio – Aerobic Relationship

There are two types of energy systems in our body: Aerobic and Anaerobic.

In the aerobic energy system, muscles get to use the oxygen continually, hence muscles can perform the activity for a longer duration. Cardio exercises like walking, running, etc use the aerobic energy system. Like I said earlier, the more oxygen used, the more calories burnt.

To understand the anaerobic system, let's get into the other category of workouts: **Strength Training.** Strength training is a type of exercise where you use weights as resistance to put pressure on your muscles. This allows the muscles to grow stronger over a period. Resistance can be in the form of weights or even your own body weight.

Chest press using dumbbells or doing push-ups are good examples of strength training.

Strength Training – Anaerobic Relationship

In this energy system, muscles do not get to use oxygen continually, hence muscles cannot perform the activity for a longer duration. E.g.: You can run for 30 minutes, but you cannot do squats or push-ups for five to ten minutes continuously.

I am not talking about the fitness challenges where participants do 100 push-ups at a stretch, I am talking about a routine, where you do a maximum of 20–30 push-ups in one set, without compromising form and technique. Since there is minimal oxygen consumption, sweating is minimal when you do push-ups compared to a run.

Now let us look at the pros and cons of each exercise type.

Cardio exercises will help you burn more calories and build your stamina, whereas strength training will help you build more muscle. You may not burn more calories during the strength training session as compared to a cardio session. So, should you be doing only cardio if your goal is fat loss? Read further and your perspective might change.

When you do cardio, you burn a good number of calories. But once the session is done, you don't burn any further calories. Whereas, when you do strength training, you burn fewer calories during the session compared to cardio, but once the session is done, your body continues to burn more calories for up to 48 hours, due to an effect called after-burn.

After-Burn

It's like your body burning more calories on its own. How? When you do strength training exercises, your metabolic rate increases. When you stop, it doesn't go back to resting immediately but remains elevated for a short time. The increased metabolism is linked to increased consumption of oxygen, which is required to help the body restore and return to a resting state and to bring the body temperature to normal levels. The more the oxygen consumed, the more calories burnt.

This is called **Excessive Post-Exercise Oxygen Consumption (EPOC).**

In simple language it means, whatever oxygen debt is created due to strength training exercises, the body recovers by consuming more oxygen post-exercise session.

EPOC is influenced by the intensity of your workouts, hence doing high-intensity anaerobic workouts helps in burning more calories even after workouts. EPOC is also influenced by your post-workout meals. If you eat the right meals, it helps the body with muscle recovery. Muscle is the only metabolic active tissue in your body, and your body needs to burn more calories on its own to maintain it. Hence, the more the muscle, the more calories are burnt on its own. So, your focus should be to add more muscle. More muscle also makes you feel stronger and adds to the right posture.

Exercise	Calories burnt during exercise	Calories burnt Post-Exercise
Cardio	More	Minimal
Strength training	Less	After-burn (24–36 hours)

Would you want your body to burn fat on its own? Of course!

So, you should do strength training.

Now tell me what will you choose: Cardio or Strength training?

Ideally, a mix of both makes more sense. So, if you plan to exercise four days a week, then three days of strength training and a day of cardio will be the right combination.

Progressive Overload

Riyansh is a college student who recently joined a gym to add some muscle. It was his second week when the following incident happened.

Riyansh: Add two more 10 kg plates, this is too light for me.

Trainer: But this is your second week. Riyansh, you need to go slow…

Riyansh: No no, I can do this. (He lifted the bar over his head for a shoulder press.) 1 count…2 counts…3 counts……4 counts……ahhhhhh, please hold the bar, I got a catch in my back!

His trainer took control of the bar and put it on the floor.

Riyansh suffered a bad catch in his upper back had to take rest for almost three weeks.

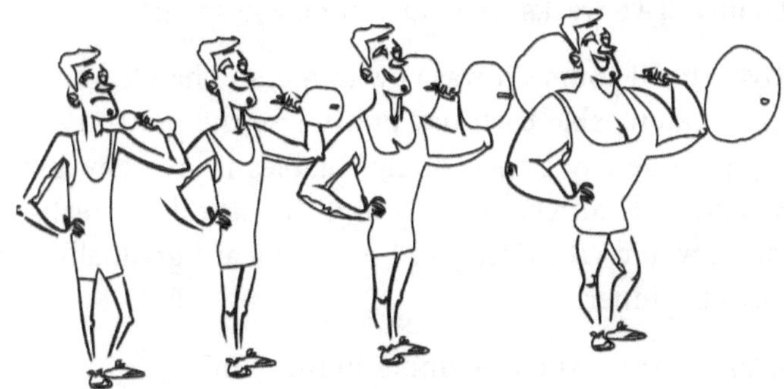

This happens with so many new gym-goers and is one of the causes of exercise injuries. I have seen this happening particularly with young guys who enthusiastically try to do something nasty and injure themselves badly just like Riyansh. Exercise injuries take time to recover and if it is related to the back/neck/shoulder it takes more time. And in the process, you lose time and interest to exercise again.

After almost a month, Riyansh met his trainer.

Riyansh: So, should we not lift heavy weights?

Trainer: Of course, you should, how else will you challenge your muscles, but there is a way to do it.

Let me explain to you a term called **Progressive Overload**.

As a kid, have you learnt the math tables?

Riyansh: Yes, I did, when I was in school.

Trainer: How did you do it?

Riyansh: I started with reciting and revising tables of 2, then 3, then 4, and in 2–3 weeks, I could do up to 15.

Trainer: Two weeks…so much time you spent?

Riyansh: Of course, it was new to me, so I had to go slow, learn a new table each day and revise the previous one. In fact, one day I tried doing 4 tables in one day, but I was not able to recollect any of it the next day. I realised that it would take time and I need to learn gradually as I was a beginner!

Trainer: Aren't you a beginner in the gym?

Riyansh: Yes, sir, I got your point. I should have listened to you and not lifted those two extra plates.

Trainer: It's not just about those two extra plates, it has more to it: your strength, your posture, the technique influences your performance. This is called **Progressive Overload**, a very important concept in the exercise world. It is a technique where you gradually increase the resistance and intensity of your exercise routine.

E.g.: In the first week of strength training, you may perform 8 repetitions at one weight. Next week, you either perform 10 -12 repetitions of the same weight or you stick to 8 repetitions and increase the weight.

But why do we need to follow this?

We need to grow and get stronger day by day. Doing the same exercises over and over and using the same weights, same intensity can put your body in a comfort zone. You may be able to lift the weight with ease, which was once challenging, but you will not see any progress in your body. When you challenge your body the right way, it may be a struggle initially, but eventually, it gives the best results.

How do we do it?

There are various ways this can be done, but before that, let's understand a few common terms:

1. **Reps** – the number of times you perform a particular exercise is called repetitions or reps. It is also called counts in common language. So, when someone says, I did 10 push-ups, he means he did 10 reps of push-ups.

2. **Sets** – a group of reps done in a row is called a set. So, a set will have X no of repetitions and there can be N number of sets. So, in the earlier example, 10 push-ups are 1 Set. Likewise, you may do 2–3 sets.

3. **Exercise Volume** – It is the number of sets done for a particular exercise routine. E.g., your chest routine can have 3 sets of push-ups, 3 sets of chest press, 2 sets of the parallel bar, and so on.

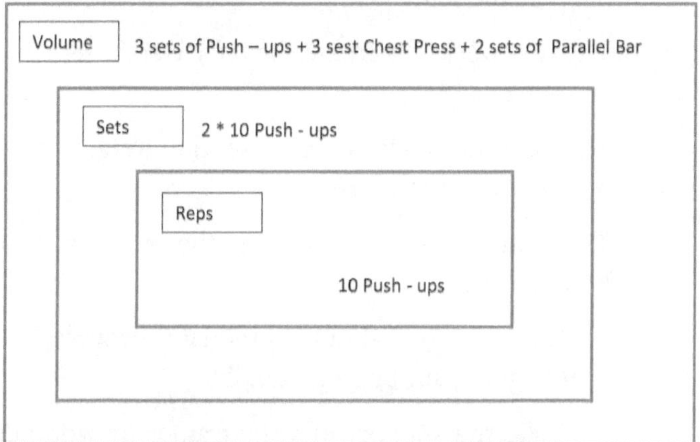

Understanding Reps, Sets and Volume

How to implement **progressive overload?**

- **Increase the reps**: In the first week, start with 6–8 reps. Check your form and if you can do it the right way, next week do 8–10 reps. This can go on increasing gradually and once you reach 10–12 reps, you need to increase the resistance rather than trying to do more.

- **Increase the weights**: First, let us understand how much is enough. It will differ from person to person. A general guideline is if you are able to do 8–10 reps using a particular weight comfortably, then that weight is not giving you good resistance and you need to add more.

  Reps and Weights go hand in hand, but as a rule of thumb, do not change both in one go. E.g., if you are increasing the reps of your shoulder press in one week, then keep the weight same; next week you can increase the weight, keeping the reps the same.

  The first week – Increase the reps; weight remains the same.

  The second week – Increase the weight; reps remain the same.

  The third week – Increase the reps, weight remains same...and so on.

  So, it is about gradual progression, challenging your body gradually.

  Take the support of your trainer or workout buddy when you start increasing the weights, so in case you lose balance, there is someone to manage it.

- **Increase the duration**: Initially, keep the duration to 15 minutes and week on week increase it by adding more sets and exercises. But restrict your overall duration to 60 mins, anything beyond that can result in fatigue and muscle loss unless you are a pro.

- **Increase the volume:** Start with 1 set of each exercise and eventually increase the volume by adding more sets and more resistance.

- **Increase the frequency**: When you start, you may do it for 2 days a week. As you settle down, you can add a day and then another one as you go ahead. But do take rest at least one day a week to help muscle recovery and gain maximum advantage from your training sessions.

- **Decrease the rest period:** In the initial days, you will need a considerably longer break between sets to recover from fatigue. But as you become regular and progress, this rest period must be minimised. Do remember what we spoke about regarding the OHR and fat burn. So, as you progress, restrict your rest period between sets to not more than 45 secs.

Include these methods as part of your exercise sessions and reap the benefits. The above rules apply to any exercise you do, including your cardio routines as well.

Warm-Up and Cool-Down

One Wednesday evening, I received a call from RK, an old friend of mine. He runs a garment store in Mumbai.

RK: I got a catch in my thigh muscle while doing a weighted squat, can you suggest a tablet for quick recovery.

Me: How did this happen, was the weight too heavy?

RK: No, it was a regular weight, I do this every week.

Me: Did u warm-up?

RK: No, I had to catch up with a friend post-workout, so wanted to finish it and rush.

Me: That is the problem RK, you missed an important ritual of a good workout.

RK: But I had missed it even before, but never got a catch.

Me: Aha… That means you have been punishing your body for long and finally, your body has reacted.

Now skip your outing and take rest for a couple of days, your body has already given you a signal and needs rest.

RK: Yes, that is what I plan to do.

Warm-up is an integral part of your workout. It makes your body physically and mentally ready for the session. Imagine, on a cold winter morning, when you go in for a shower and there is no hot water: Do you get under the water immediately? No, in fact, most will avoid taking a shower, while the brave ones like you and me will stick our finger in first, then hand, and then the entire body. Why do we do that? By putting the finger in first, our body gets an idea about the temperature of the water and it starts preparing itself, then when we put our hand in, our body is ready to embrace the cold water and it gives us the confidence to jump in. Now, if someone pushes you into this cold water suddenly, imagine the kind of shock you would get.

That is how your body reacts when you miss a warm-up and directly start with a set of squats *(or any other exercises)*.

Some of the benefits of warm-up:

- It increases the blood flow and oxygen supply to the muscles, which gives them the required stability and nourishment before getting into an intense workout.

- It improves the range of motion allowing your joints to move fully.

- It warms up the muscles which help in removing stiffness, making it easy to work out.

How do you warm-up:

Rotate all your joints clockwise and anticlockwise for 10 reps preferably in the following sequence:

- Shoulder

- Waist

- Ankle

- Neck

- Elbows

- Wrist

Next, focus on increasing the heart rate by adding an element of cardio as follows:

- Jog on the spot

- Skip

- High Knees

- Mummy Kicks

- Jumping Jacks

- Sprints

Fifteen reps of each are good enough to rev up your heart rate and body temperature too. Those suffering from knee or ankle pain, should avoid jumps and replace them with variations *(different exercises)*. E.g.: Skipping can be replaced with marching on the spot. Jumping jacks can be replaced with plain jacks, etc.

Do refer to the warm-up video in the Appendix.

Once you do these 2 sequences, then you are good to start with your main exercise sequence as per your plan. Once you complete the main exercise sequence, your need to do the concluding part: Cool-down.

Cool-Down

You have used your muscles extensively; your heart rate and body temperature have gone up during the session. Now, as you end the session, you need to relax your muscles by stretching them and also bring the body temperature and heart rate to normal.

Imagine your exercise session as some kind of box in space. To get into it, you have to make yourself ready *(Warm-up)* so you get permission to go there. Similarly, to come out of it and return to this planet, you again need to get ready *(Cool-down)*, so you get the required permission. If you miss out on any of it, there are chances you may get stuck in space, just like our own PK (movie).

It has been observed that cool-down is the most ignored part and is often skipped for lack of awareness and time.

I was taking my Wednesday morning session and it was a core day. I had almost finished the workout and had given the last break to start the cool-down session.

Vivan, a software engineer had joined our fitness programme, a couple of days ago.

As the workout session was about to end, he put the following message on chat:

Vivan: I have to leave for work, so I need to log off now.

Me: We still have to cool-down, finish it and then leave.

Vivan: I am getting late for work.

Me: Do you not want to reap maximum benefits from this session, or do you want to get up tomorrow morning with some pain? This will not take more than five minutes.

Vivan: Okay. (He completed the cool-down sequence.)

I often get these kinds of requests from our new participants. The old ones (*in terms of association with us)* don't do that.

Some of the benefits of Cool-down:

Normalise the heart rate – As you finish the workout, you want your heart rate to return to normal slowly. This helps you avoid light-headedness or a feeling of faintness.

Regulates breathing – When your heart rate increases with the workout, breathing becomes deeper. A cool-down session allows your breathing to gradually return to normal.

Prevents injuries – Your muscles have really worked hard (*stretched, pulled*) during the session and they need to be relaxed till they are warm to avoid injuries. This also helps to increase the range of motion in the joints, which increases the overall flexibility.

How do you cool-down?

The focus should be to primarily stretch the muscle groups which have been used for the workout session. E.g., when you do an upper-body sequence, you may want to focus more on the chest, shoulder, triceps, and forearm muscles, but you should also look at stretching the overall body.

This needs to be followed by a 2–3-minute breathing or meditation session. This really helps to cool-down your body and mind.

So, this is the right sequence: Warm-up + Main exercises + Cool-down.

Do refer to the cool-down videos in Appendix.

Muscle Soreness Post-Exercise

Umang, a lawyer by profession had joined our fitness programme a week earlier, and he was a beginner. We had accordingly given him the exercise routine to get him started. He did well in the first session, doing minimal reps and taking adequate rest. When I checked with him in the evening, which is our normal practice, he was all fine. But I was aware that he'd experience some pain when he woke up the next day.

That was when he sent me this message.

Umang: I am skipping today's session as am feeling weak and my body is paining.

Me: It is a part of the process and you should be fine in a day.

It also shows you had a good workout session. Rest today and just go for a walk in the evening for 15–20 minutes and you will feel better. See you in the next class.

Umang: But I followed your instructions only, so why this pain.

Me: Let me explain the concept of **Muscle soreness and DOMS** to you.

DOMS or Delayed Onset Muscle Soreness is a muscle-related pain that normally begins 12- 24 hours after a workout session. Restricted range of motion, drop in muscle strength, muscle pain are the typical symptoms. Of these, muscle pain is the most common.

Body akad gaya, is what people normally say. (My body has become stiff.)

You feel this pain when you touch that particular muscle and gently press it to experience the pain. I call this *sweet pain,* something you enjoy because it reminds you that you have started doing workouts. This pain does not cause much discomfort as such, but you know it is there. It stays for a day or 2 and slowly goes away.

Taking rest, going for a walk, taking a hot bath has been found to effectively relieve DOMS. It has also been observed that if you stretch well *(cool-down)* post-workout, the intensity of DOMS goes down.

DOMS vs Exercise Injury

DOMS will settle down gradually. But if it goes beyond 3–4 days and it is causing you a lot of discomfort in doing your daily activities, then it can be a case of injury. Exercise injuries can take time to heal, depending on their type. Rest and proper treatment need to be taken.

I observed Nikhil as he did push-ups.

Me: Why are you not doing a full push-up?

Nikhil: I have pain in my triceps muscle, so I cannot do it.

Me: Since when?

Nikhil: It has been two weeks now.

Me: Did you not take a break?

Nikhil: No no, I cannot miss my exercise, I am going on vacation next week, I need a beach body.

Me: But you are doing it wrong, further damaging the muscle, which can be severe.

Nikhil: That is ok, I have been taking pain killers and will take a break after I come back.

Me: What if this pain becomes worse when you are flaunting your beach body?

Nikhil: I did not think about it, should I take a break?

Me: Yes, it will help you in the long run.

Let's Talk about Exercise Injuries

There is always a give and take relationship with your body. You take care of your body by doing exercises and eating good food, your body responds by becoming stronger and getting in good shape. But if you overexert and do not give it the much-needed rest, it will respond accordingly. In fact, pain is the way our body tells us to rest, and you need to respect that message and act accordingly. If you do that, it will heal gradually. If you don't, the pain and injury will grow and will not allow you to do your daily routine, forget exercise.

You would have read about how the careers of many athletes and sportspersons ended due to injuries. I have seen many examples in gyms where people have worked out despite pain and have literally been out of exercise for 6–9 months. The josh and adrenaline rush will always push you to work out, but you need to take a conscious call.

Exercise injuries can happen to anyone, right from beginners to seasoned athletes. Chances of it happening to beginners are more as they are not in control of their form and technique, whereas an athlete will manage it well.

Missing the warm-up and cool-down are one of the main reasons for exercise injures.

The most common exercise injuries are:

- Shoulder injury

- Ankle sprain

- Wrist pain

- Back and neck strain

Can it be avoided? Yes.

How?

- Focus on your form and technique.

- Do not overdo, follow the principle of Progressive Overload.

- Never miss warm-up and cool-down.

- Eat a right pre- and post-workout meal.

- Do not work out in pain, take rest.

- Listen and respect your body signals.

- Take care of your troublesome areas, everyone has that.

How to treat workout injuries?

- Take rest.

- Use the hot/cold treatment.

- Apply compression bandage.

- See a doctor.

DOMS	Exercise Injuries
Soreness 12–24 hours post-workout	Soreness at the beginning and end of workout
Burning, aching sensation when muscles are engaged	Sharp, unbearable pains at all time
Last from 1–3 days	Last longer, until treated
Improves with stretching, rest and few aerobic exercises	Worsens with stretching and exercises

How to start post-injury

1. Take a break till you recover from pain – never exercise in pain. (*Forget No Pain, No Gain.*) Once the pain has stopped, start with isolation exercises to strengthen the muscles *(Use free or light weights. Using resistance bands also help.)*

2. After a week, check how the body responds. *(There will be DOMS for one or two days, which is normal.)*

3. If there is no pain, increase the weights/reps. *(Go slow, do not be overly enthusiastic and lift heavy weights. Appreciate that your body is responding positively.)*

4. Do it for two to three weeks and slowly get back to your regular workout routine.

5. If you experience pain again, go back to step 1.

Exercise Meals

"Don't eat for one hour, post-workout," Garry told his friend as he got down from the treadmill.

"Is it," asked his friend?

"Yes, if you don't eat, your body will burn fat stores to get the required energy. This will help you lose more weight."

"That's a good tip."

"I have been following this rule, intentionally not eating before and after my workouts, and see how much weight I have lost."

One of the gym trainers who stood close by interrupted to tell him that he had lost muscle not fat! "If you do not eat the right workout meals, you are just wasting your time in the gym," he added.

Garry was shocked. "What do you mean by that?"

"I can see that you have lost weight, but tell me, do you feel strong?" the trainer asked.

Gary kept quiet.

"You are losing muscle as you are not eating the required meals. Hence, you don't feel very strong," the trainer added.

"Can you tell me more about workout meals?" asked Gary.

"Sure," said the trainer.

Our health is dependent on the food choices we make. Similarly, our workouts and results depend a lot on what we consume before, during, and after the workout session. If this is not managed well, then the time and the efforts we spend on exercise are of no value.

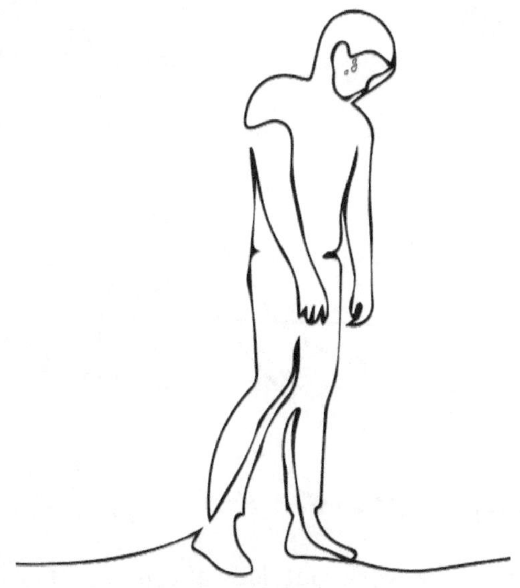

"Oh, I have been doing this for almost four months now. No wonder, I don't feel my muscles growing," Gary said, looking at his 12-inch ka biceps.

Let's look at exercise meals. It's basically a 3-course meal:

Pre-workout meals – What you eat before the workout influences your energy levels and performance. If you have not eaten the right food, you may experience a drop in your energy, leading to poor form or quitting the session.

Working on an empty stomach is like driving a bike on reserve fuel. You will never know when it will break down.

What are the options?

Have 3–4 medium-size dates or 2 bananas at least 15 minutes before the workout.

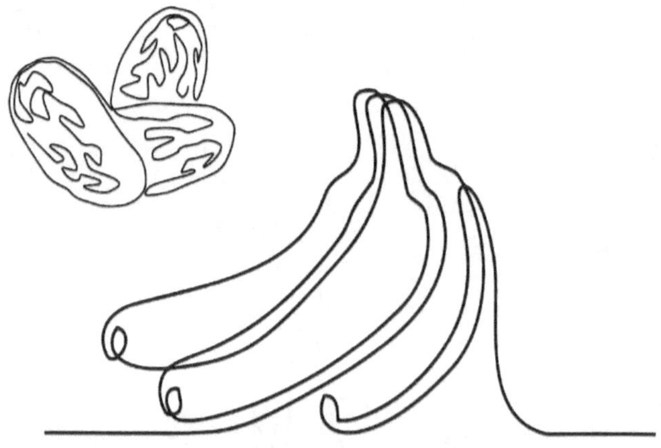

If you plan to work out late afternoon, then keep a gap of at least two hours after lunch. You should avoid any heavy food before the workout as it will restrict the blood flow to the working muscles and impact performance.

During Workout Meals – We lose water and energy through sweat during a workout session and keeping ourselves hydrated is a must. Sip water at regular intervals.

Post-Workout Meals – This is where most go wrong. The time frame of 45 mins post-workout is called the magical window and if you feed your body the right nutrition during this period, you reap maximum benefits from the workout session. Protein forms the main element of this meal as it aids muscle recovery. If this meal is missed, you do not get any benefits from your workout session.

What are the options?

Five minutes post-workout: Have a seasonal fruit.

Fifteen minutes post-workout: Have a protein-rich meal, preferably a whey protein shake. Alternatives are eggs, paneer, mushroom-based meals.

Ninety minutes post-workout: Have a balanced meal. Chapati/Roti + Dal + Veggies or any home-cooked balanced meal are good options.

Eating a fruit post-workout helps in replenishing glycogen stores and regulates blood sugar levels. It also creates an environment in your body to absorb the next protein-rich meal. A whey protein shake with the required amino acids helps in the recovery of muscles. Being in liquid format, it gets absorbed quickly unlike the solid sources of protein and starts its repair work immediately. A balanced meal is the right combination of protein, carbs, and fats. We will talk more about it in the Meals chapter.

Isolation vs Compound

Uff, take it quickly, I cannot hold my breath further, said Birdy, while posing for a picture of his bulging biceps and trying to cover his paunch with a bag at the same time.

When your goal is to reduce overall body fat, you cannot just do bicep curls.

I am not saying they are bad, but your focus should be on doing **compound exercises** like squats, deadlifts, bench press, etc, that work on multiple muscle groups at the same time. Squats work on quadriceps, glutes, and claves together.

On a funny note: You cannot flex your biceps with a paunch hiding in your backyard.

Isolation exercises work on a single muscle group at a time and work best when strengthening a certain muscle group.

When your goal is to get lean and reduce fat, compound exercises help in the optimum involvement of multiple muscle groups, which helps burn more calories, improves muscular coordination, elevates heart rate (fat burn) and improves strength and flexibility.

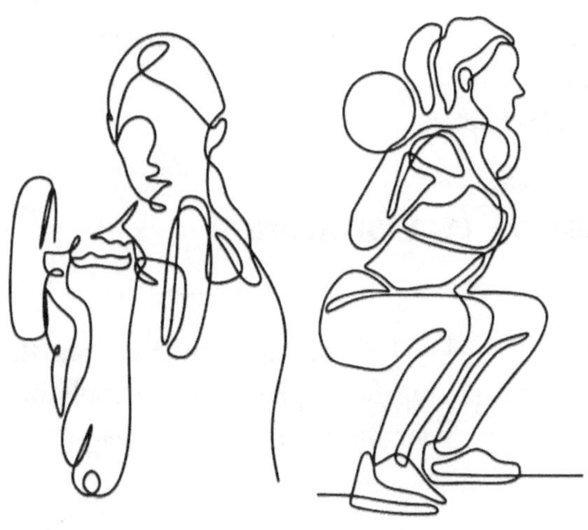

Should we only do compound exercises?

Seventy per cent of your strength training time can be allocated for compound and rest for isolation exercises. Isolation exercises also offer benefits in terms of strengthening a single muscle, with more focus on providing more definition to a particular area, e.g., bicep curls, tricep kickbacks, crunches, etc. Initially, do more compound exercises to lose body fat and then as you progress, focus on the specific area through isolation exercises.

HIIT

10 burpees + 12 straight punches + 20 jumping jacks + 30 sec plank hold. Break.

Repeat till fatigue.

If this sequence excites you, then you can hit your fat stores with HIIT.

HIIT or High-Intensity Interval Training is a set of workouts that involve short periods of intense exercises alternated with brief recovery periods. Basically, an exercise after exercise with minimal rest. This works very well for fat loss and also allows you to finish your workout in a short time, rather than doing those slow workouts for 60 minutes, which can be boring for a few and may not add much value.

Benefits of HIIT

- First, it elevates heart rate and we have been talking about the relation between elevated heart rate and fat loss.

- It helps you burn more calories. *(After-burn effect.)*

- It works on the principle of compound workouts, as it involves many movements using multiple muscle groups.

- It complements your fat and weight loss journey.

- It also allows you to test your strength and stamina and gives you a feeling of *deja vu* when you see such improvements in your strength and agility.

- And finally, it makes your workouts interesting, giving you the required josh and adrenaline rush and a sense of satisfaction when you complete the workout.

There is absolutely no limit to mixing your workouts based on compound and HIIT. But keep these few things in mind:

- Do higher intensity before lower-intensity exercises. *(Burpees before chest press.)*

- Cover bigger muscles before the smaller muscles (*Leg muscles before biceps.)*

- Push yourself to complete the circuit.

- If you feel breathless or experience pain or a catch, stop immediately and rest.

Male vs Female Exercises

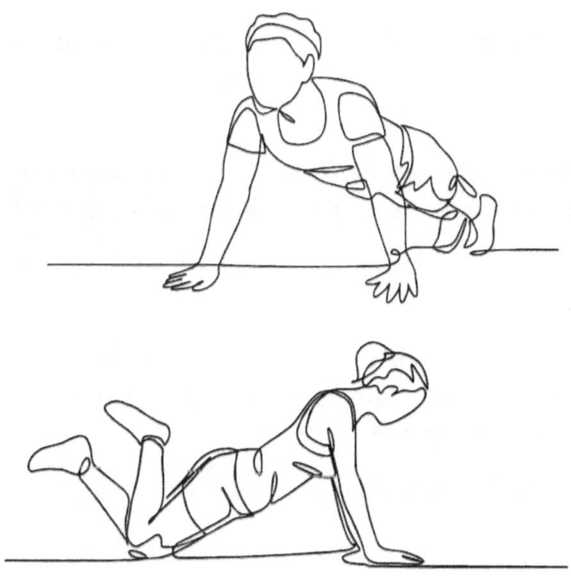

Sangeeta, a housewife had come for a consulting session. She wanted to lose her post-maternity weight. We discussed the types of exercises we do, and I showed her a few videos of our sessions. She scrolled through a few videos, trying to understand how we do it. As she scrolled down further, she was surprised to see a video where Prita and Artha were doing advanced burpees.

Sangeeta: Yeh to ladkla log ka exercise hai, muzhe aisi body nahi banani hai, sirf thoda weight loss karna hai, (These exercises are meant for guys. I just want to lose some weight.)

Me: Aisa kuch alag exercises nahi hota hai, I replied in the same tone. (There are no such gender-separate exercises.)

Sangeeta: Hota hai na, maine padha hai Google pe: special exercises for women. (I know, there are women-specific exercises).

Then I showed her a few of the workout videos of our other female participants and she was surprised.

Sangeeta: Yeh sab mai bhi kar sakti hoo? (Will I be able to do all these exercises?)

Me: Of course, ek bar start ho jayega, then gradually tumhara strength badhega (Just start and you will build the required strength).

Sangeeta: I want to do it.

There is this misconception that certain workouts are only for men and women cannot do them. Over the past few years, I have seen so many women doing amazing workouts, right from intense HIITs to heavy strength training. So, your gender does not determine your exercises, your goal does. If you are looking for fat loss and building a good body, then all that is mentioned above holds good for you. Just go ahead and do your squats, lunges, deadlifts, burpees, bench press, etc. Trust me, you will not look like a bodybuilder, which most females fear, but you will look amazing strong, and fit.

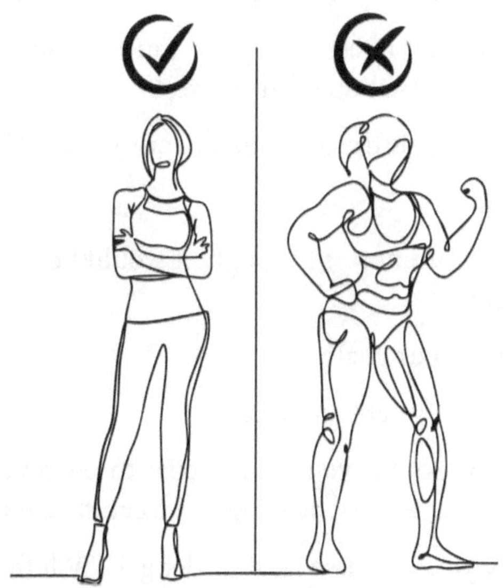

There are some differences in strength and other parameters between the two genders, like men can lift more weight, whereas women are generally more flexible, but these do not impact your exercise performance and your goal.

REST

Sagar was about to get married and was desperate to lose weight. That's when he got in touch with me through some reference.

Sagar: I need to work out on all days, not just four days a week. Can you give me that?

Me: For beginners, we do four days a week, then we add the 5th and 6th day if needed.

Sagar: But I need to lose weight and I cannot miss a day.

Me: You need to rest too, your muscles do not grow when you exercise but when you rest.

Sagar: Ok, what is the duration of your workout?

Me: 45 minutes.

Sagar: Just 45 minutes? I thought it would be at least give 60–90 minutes.

Me: What is your goal?

Sagar: To lose weight and look fit.

Me: This works for you, take a trial tomorrow, and get back with your experience. Then, we can take it forward.

Sagar: Are you sure, isse farak padenga? (Will this help?)

Me: A hundred per cent padenga, do not worry.

And that is how his journey started.

If you are someone who says, I want to work out every single day, you are not doing your body any good. Rest allows your muscles to rebuild and grow. More the muscles, more the calorie burn, more the fat loss. Taking enough rest also reduces the chances of injury.

When you are a beginner, exercise on alternate days: M-W-F and take rest on other days. As you progress, add a day more, but ensure that you don't exercise for more than four consecutive days, without taking rest. Once you are a complete pro, you can even do six days a week and have at least one day of rest.

Overtraining also puts stress on your body, disturbing your mental health. One last thing, taking rest gives you time for family and hobbies, enhances your mood, and makes you ready for the next session.

Breathing Techniques

Breathe normally: The most effective way to breathe during strength training is to inhale as you lower the resistance *(weight)* and exhale as you lift the weight. You should never hold your breath, as it might lead to an increase in your blood pressure.

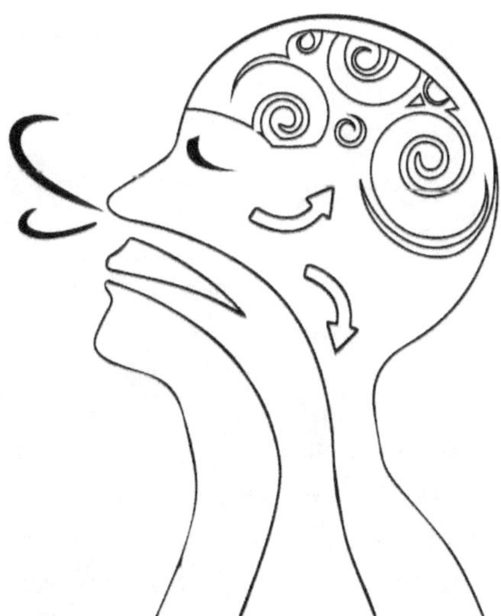

Practice this 4-7-8 rule to improve your breathing pattern:

- Exhale completely through your mouth, making a whoosh sound.

- Close your mouth and inhale quietly through your nose to a mental count of four.

- Hold your breath for a count of seven.

- Exhale completely through your mouth, making a whoosh sound to a count of eight.

Are you stuck?

I have hit a plateau, is the most common phrase you will hear across gyms.

What it means is, my body is not responding to exercise and not showing results.

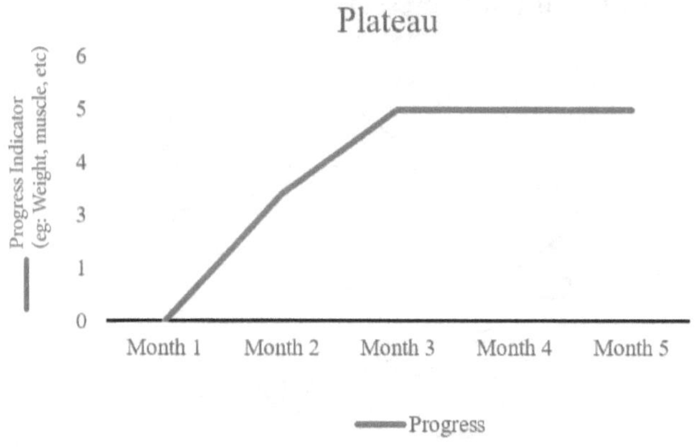

When you exercise regularly, you start seeing results and it motivates you further. However, as time passes, your body adjusts to the exercises and your progress slows down. E.g.: In the first two months, you were able to lose a considerable amount of fat and inches off your waistline. Now, suddenly, you feel that it is not moving forward.

There can be various reasons for this. I will highlight a few of them:

- Overtraining and not taking the required rest.

- Not following the principle of progressive overload. *(Not challenging your body)*

- Not eating the right way. *(Pre-workout – during workout – post-workout)*

There are ways in which you can break this plateau:

- Take rest for a week.

- Change your exercise routine, try something different for two weeks.

- Eat five to six portion-controlled meals a day.

- Drink more water.

- Manage stress well.

- And last and most important, look at your fitness goal, feel charged up, and start again with zeal.

Have rocking workouts and build a body you always dreamt of.

Now that we are clear about the topic of exercise, let's look at an equally important topic: Meals.

Chapter 8
Managing Your Meals

Raman has been a regular gym-goer for three years. He does heavy strength training and likes to wear fitting tees to flaunt his biceps and broad shoulders. As such he looks fit, but in those tees, his love handles, and paunch are visible. He has tried working on them for long but was not able to get results.

"This is dam tasty," said Raman, while taking a big bite of a double cheeseburger.

"How do you manage to stay fit by eating all this junk," asked his friend?

"Eat – Burn – Eat is my funda. (logic)."

"What does that mean," asked his friend?

Eat whatever you want and burn the same by exercising. And then he gave many examples of how he does heavy workouts and burns calories.

This is not just in the case of Raman. There are many who believe the same. And it is absolutely wrong for the following reason: One session of strength training will help you burn around 200 calories, whereas one double cheeseburger has at least 750 calories, of which almost 50% come from fat. It's not just the number of calories on the higher side, but their source is also not right (50% from fat).

So, **Calories Burnt** < **Calories Consumed** + 50% calories from fat.

Results: Fat gain.

Hence what you eat is equally or I would say more important than what you burn.

Let's talk about Meal Planning. Just like we plan our vacations and work to get the desired outcomes, we need to plan our meals to get the desired results. The first and foremost thing is to recollect what we've learnt in school: The size of our stomach is the size of our fist. So, the food we eat must be in the same proportion.

Now imagine, that the walls of our stomach are made of an elastic material and it will expand in proportion to the food we put in it. It can expand as much.

The problem is it does not contract on its own ☺.

So, we need to ensure that we give it the required quantity of food, which is also known as **Portion Control.**

This term is often used in the fitness world and what it means is eating the required serving of food in one meal. It is better to have five to six portion-controlled meals throughout the day, rather than two to three big meals. When we do that, we don't overeat in one meal. If you have the habit of eating only two to three meals, you tend to eat more. Why? Our system is much smarter than we think. We talk about Artificial Intelligence, but we don't appreciate the human body and the way it functions.

When we eat fewer meals, our system thinks that it has only two to three opportunities throughout the day to get food and it fears that if it doesn't eat more, then it might starve as there are big gaps between meals. E.g.: If you are a person who eats breakfast at 8:00 a.m., lunch at 1:00 p.m., and dinner at 9:00 p.m., your system has adjusted to this eating pattern. It knows that it will get food only at these time intervals and accordingly it demands food and gets into a cycle of heavy eating.

Whereas, when you have 5–6 portion-controlled meals, you pass a message to your system that it will get food at regular intervals and the system responds by adjusting to the smaller portions, as it is aware that it will soon get its next supply of nutrition. Also, this gives time for our stomach to digest well. There are different ways to measure how much is enough, but the best way is to listen to your stomach as it does give a signal when it›s full. Right from eating slowly to what you are eating, it matters a lot.

We will talk more about digestion in a separate chapter. For now, let us look at how to plan these meals.

Like I said in one of the chapters when you sleep your body still needs the energy to do the repair work and it comes from the food you eat. When you wake up, your body craves more energy and you need to provide it, rather than starving it. It has already starved for seven to eight hours and now is expecting the right food.

Hence as soon as you wake up and are done with your morning chores, have a glass of water and a few dry fruits. Soak black raisins and almonds overnight. This works very well for this meal. It gives you the much-needed dose of energy. *Water can also be consumed immediately after waking up.*

First Meal: Water + Dry fruits (4–5 soaked black raisins + 2 almonds)

To be taken within 15 mins of waking up.

Post this, you may want to check your messages, emails, news, etc. What is preferred next is spending five to ten minutes doing deep breathing exercises to refresh your mind. This can be done preferably in an open space or by keeping your windows open. Trust me, this makes your mind fresh and sets a positive tone for the day. Once you are done with this, it's time to have the most important meal of your day: **Breakfast.**

Breakfast or break–ur–fast is the much-needed meal for your body and you need to plan it well. Before getting into details, let us understand a few things about your Macros and Micros (Macronutrients and Micronutrients). You may have heard these terms often, now let's talk about it.

The word macro means larger quantities: Carbohydrates, Proteins, Fats are major components of our meals.

And micro means smaller quantities: Vitamins and Minerals play an important role.

I am not going to elaborate much on this, as there are umpteen resources available. The only thing I would highlight, is we need all of them as part of our meals.

You read it right, we will also need fats (good fats) and carbs (good carbs).

- Carbs are a good source of energy; hence they are also included as part of a pre-workout meal.

- Protein acts as a muscle builder and hence is included as part of a post-workout meal.

- Fats protect our organs and help in keeping our body warm.

These will vary based on your goals.

Hence, we cannot remove any of them from our meals. It needs to be in the following proportion:

- Carbs – 40–45%

- Protein – 30–40%

- Fats – 25–30%

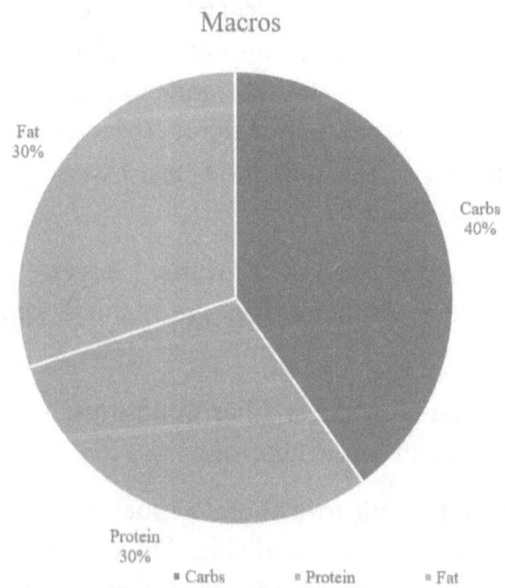

You can also read it the other way:

- Almost 40–45% of your calories should come from good carbs.

- Almost 30–45% from lean protein, and

- Not more than 25–30% from good fats.

Carbs

They are our central source of food. If you look at the food you've consumed from childhood till now, you will realise that majority of it is carbs, because of its easy availability and the energy it gives your body.

Look at how we start our day: Poha, upma, idli, chapati, paratha, breads, oats, etc, they all have carbs. Also, breakfast made from poha keeps you full for longer compared to biscuits and cookies. If you get the right amount of energy from carbs, then it prevents the protein from being used as energy, and let it do its main function of muscle building.

It has been found that good carbs help in your reflex action and managing mood swings too.

Despite these benefits, carbs have earned a bad reputation that it makes you fat and hence most do not consume it regularly (no carb or low carbs meals).

Like any other food group, there are foods rich in good carbs and foods rich in bad carbs.

Good ones:

- Starchy vegetables

- Rice (brown)

- Oatmeal

- Chapati, Roti, Paratha

- Pulses

- Whole wheat bread

- Fruits

- Milk

- Chana

- Nuts

- Salads

Bad ones:

- White bread

- Biscuits

- Cookies

- Pizza

- Burgers

- Ice creams

- Chocolates

- Jellies

- Doughnuts

- Aerated beverages

- Fries

- Chips

What is so different between the two groups of carbs?

Good carbs like poha and chapati take more time to digest and hence keep you full for long, whereas bad carbs like cookies get digested quickly, creating a sugar rush and making you feel hungry sooner, resulting in overeating. Good carbs like fruits, grains, and vegetables also have fibre which helps in the digestion process. We will talk more about fibre in a later chapter. Meals that include oatmeal, sweet potatoes, bananas, brown rice contain a good amount of tryptophan, which helps in getting sound sleep.

Bad carbs are low in nutrition, have bad calories and trans-fat which leads to obesity. Regular consumption of bad fats leads to lifestyle diseases like diabetes, blood pressure, heart issues, and many other issues. Now you know the reason behind your paunch is not just being sedentary, but also regular consumption of burgers, cookies, chips, etc.

Food is not always bad. The way you cook it can also influence its nutritional value. E.g.: Potato is a good source, but you make chips out of it, then you know it is not healthy. The same is the case with carrot and carrot ka halwa (gajar ka halwa). It is not required that you completely abandon the bad ones, but ensure that they are consumed sparingly (can be part of your cheat meal, which we will talk about it later).

Protein

They are muscle builders and like we discussed, to maintain muscles, the body needs to expend calories, aiding fat loss. A lot of research has shown that consuming the right amount of protein-rich meals keeps you full (panner sandwich vs cookies). It also helps the immune system stay strong.

Post-workout, imagine that your muscles are broken down just like hair splits. When you consume protein-rich food, it reaches these damaged muscles and helps them recover. Hence, it is required to have protein-rich food post-workout. Lack of protein will not allow the recovery of muscles and will negate the benefits of your workout. Also, its shortage creates a lot of flab in the body leading to obesity.

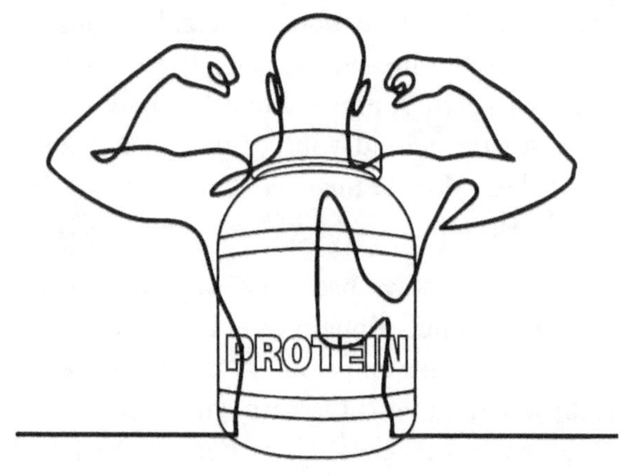

How much protein is needed?

A sedentary individual needs 1 gram of protein per kg of their body weight and the ones who exercise regularly need 1.2 to 1.5 grams per kg of their body weight daily.

E.g.: If my body weight is 70 kgs, then:

I would need a minimum of 70 grams of protein.

And if I am active, I need 84 to 105 grams every single day.

Recollect how to check your ideal body weight, and consume protein accordingly.

Bhavesh runs a grocery store in the eastern suburbs of Mumbai. Due to the sedentary nature of his work, he had gained a lot of weight. He wanted to exercise and get fit and that's when he got in touch with me. We discussed his meal plan during which the topic of protein consumption came up.

Bhavesh: I am a vegetarian, hence cannot consume a lot of protein.

Me: There are a lot of vegetarian sources to take care of your protein needs.

Bhavesh: But my friends always say that there are no options.

Me: Actually, people attribute protein to non-veg food, but this is not the case. There are many options available.

Bhavesh: Is it, then tell me more about it?

Me: Here you go.

Where is protein?

It is present in both vegetarian and animal sources and can be consumed accordingly.

Vegetarian sources:

- Cottage cheese (paneer)
- Pulses (also are a source of carbohydrates)
- Sprouts
- Lentils (dal)
- Green peas
- Mixed seeds (pumpkin, sunflower, etc.)
- Kidney beans (rajma)
- Chickpeas
- Peanuts
- Soy n soy products
- Tofu
- Nuts (almonds, walnuts, macadamia)
- Yogurt
- Peanut butter
- Milk
- Flax seeds, chia seeds

Non-vegetarian sources:

- Chicken
- Turkey
- Fish
- Eggs
- Red Meat

Many plant-based proteins are not complete proteins, but when they are combined with good carbs, they create the right effect.

E.g. Rice and rajma when consumed together make a complete protein.

Bhavesh: Rajma – bhaat maru priy che (Rajma and rice are my favourites)

Fats

Kaata hi kaate ko nikalta hai. (Use a thorn to remove a thorn).

This is so true about fats. There are various benefits of fats, but the one I'd like to highlight is that good fats help eliminate bad fats. Not all fats are bad, and the good ones are needed by our body. Fat allows us to store energy, provide cushion to our vital organs, and also adds flavour and texture to our food.

"Hum usko accha vitamin wala khana khilate hai, per uske body ko lagta hi nhai hai, dekho kitna dubla patla ho gaya hai yeh." (We feed vitamin-rich foods to our kid, still, he is not healthy.)

Have you heard this before? I keep hearing this from every other mom. (You know mothers always think their kids are not fat ☺.) Jokes apart, what she means is that her kid's body is not ready to absorb these vitamins. Good fats play an important role here. One of its functions is to absorb fat-soluble vitamins. And in the absence of fat, these vitamins are not used by the body.

Now you know the reason behind it: *Mere body ko lagta nahi. (It doesn't help my body) Start having good fats, phir sab lagega. (Then it will help.)*

We all know examples of bad fats:

Bad Fats:

- French fries
- Doughnuts
- Cookies
- Sour cream
- Cream biscuits
- Aerated beverages
- Pakoras
- Butter
- Chips
- Wada Pav
- Samosa
- Ice cream

And the list contains all that we classify as junk.

As I said, not all fats are bad, let's look at the good ones.

Good Fats:

- Walnuts
- Coconut
- Ghee
- Nuts
- Eggs

- Curd

- Beans

- Fish

- Cold-pressed oils

- Tofu

- Nut butter

- Dark chocolate

- Groundnuts

Start adding good fats to your meals regularly and see how it helps you.

Let's go back to Bhavesh.

Bhavesh: I also get sweet cravings post-lunch/dinner and I tend to eat sweets or chocolates. This has made me put on a lot of weight.

Me: This is a common problem and is one of the leading causes of obesity.

Bhavesh: How do I manage it, is there any replacement for sweets?

Me: Yes, there are. Add good fats like ghee and coconut to your meals, your cravings will be reduced.

Bhavesh: Isn't ghee fattening?

Me: Absolutely not, start consuming it and get back with your feedback.

Special mention of ghee is required here, as in the past it had earned a bad reputation and was out of most kitchens. But it has amazing health benefits, over and above adding flavour to your food. Ensure that you make it a part of your daily meals.

How much to eat?

One thumb rule: Add ghee in a way it adds flavour to your food but ensure that it doesn't supersede the original taste. You can have one spoon a day over your dal, rice, chapati, roti, etc.

One last thing, there are some fats which are added to food to increase their shelf life and are considered as the worst type of fat. They are mostly found in processed foods like cookies, cakes, chips, and should be avoided.

They not only add to the bad cholesterol but also lower the good cholesterol. Since they are mostly found in packed foods, reading food labels to understand the nutritional value is important. We have one chapter dedicated to reading nutrition labels.

Vitamins and Minerals

When you hear Vitamins and Minerals, you feel healthy. Isn't it? They are called Micros and are required in smaller quantities than Macros. They play various roles, right from building our immune system, to taking care of our skin, protecting our bones, teeth, and much more.

Check your D3, your doctor will tell you when you go in for back pain.

Your D3 is low, you need to take Vitamin D3 shots/ supplements. Also, go for a walk around 7–7.30 am, thoda pet bhi kam ho jayega (Your stomach will go in) and you will get natural D3.

How many have heard this?

Though these micros are required in tiny amounts, their absence can cause a lot of issues and the most common is a deficiency of vitamin D3, causing neck and back pain.

Micros are available from food sources and also in the form of supplements. Ensure that they are consumed in the required quantities.

With this brief knowledge about macros and micros, let's go back to meal planning and ensure that both macros and micros are included as part of meals.

We discussed that the first meal should be the following:

First Meal: Water + Dry fruits (4–5 soaked black raisins + 2 almonds)

To be taken within 15 mins of waking up.

Let us move ahead to the next and the most important meal of the day: Breakfast.

As I said, what you eat for breakfast sets the tone for your day. If you eat healthily, you will have an energetic and agile day, whereas when you start with junk, you feel sluggish over and above feeling guilty.

Go back to your experience and think about how you felt when you ate those dense chocolate cookies for breakfast. You would have felt amazing while eating them for sure, but what happened 30 minutes later... GUILT! And now think about how energetic your mornings were when you had poha or upma for breakfast.

What makes a good breakfast? A meal that is a combination of good carbs, protein, and good fats with a touch of vitamins and minerals.

Second Meal: Breakfast

Options: One boiled egg or 2 pieces of panner + any one of the below

Have this meal within the first hour of the day.

- One chapati + veggies

- One dosa (any available batter) + Chutney/ Sambhar

- Two idlis + chutney

- Oatmeal + 1 banana

- Uttapa

- Poha

- Upma

- Brown bread with lots of veggies (sandwich)

- One moong dal chilla

- One homemade thalipeeth with curd

- Paneer Burji + 1 brown/multigrain bread toast/1 chapati

- Egg omelette/egg boiled/scrambled egg + 2 slices of multigrain bread/1 chapati.

How many of you think that eating healthy can be expensive?

You can make simple changes to existing meals to make them balanced and nutritious. Let us take the example of the most common breakfast food: Poha.

Poha as you know is a carbohydrate, so how do we make it a balanced meal?

- Add sprouted moong/peanuts, grated panner as a source of protein.

- Add grated coconut as a source of good fat.

- Add pomegranate as a source of vitamins and fibre.

- Just squeeze lime and enjoy your meal.

Such changes do not need much effort and are cost-effective. They work very well in terms of adding the required nutrition to your meals.

Similarly, you can make your preferred breakfast foods (upma, idli, paratha, etc) healthy and have a great start to your day.

Your next meal called **mid-meal** sits between breakfast and lunch and works well by giving you a small dose of energy and reduces gaps between meals.

Third Meal: A good time to have it 1.5–2 hours after breakfast and the options are as follows:

- Fruit

- Handful of nuts

- Chiki with no sugar (jaggery based)

- Cup of Chana/Singdana/Makahana/Corn

- Soups

Have this meal and you will have fewer cravings and probably a lighter lunch. If you are working, you can carry fruit or keep snacks like chana, singdana in your drawer. If you are someone whose work involves travel, then this can be conveniently carried in your bag.

I discussed with Akriti, a social media content manager about her untimely meals and how they affected her health. Her work schedules keep her busy in the first half of the day and her lunch is had mostly after 3:00 p.m.

Akriti: I get so hungry by the time I have lunch, that I end up hogging.

Me: What time do you have breakfast?

Akriti: Once I reach the office, around 9:00 a.m.

Me: There is a big gap between your breakfast and lunch, you need to add a mid-meal around 11:30 a.m.

Akriti: Ohh, that's peak time, and I am mostly in meetings. It would not look good to eat in front of everyone.

Me: Can't you take a five-minute break to eat a fruit or a few nuts?

Akriti – Will that suffice?

Me: It will manage your hunger pangs and will help you eat a lighter lunch.

Akriti – I will give it a try.

How many of you have this concern? First thing, you know that you are focusing on your fitness and your body needs food at regular intervals, so you should have it. It takes less than five minutes for this meal, and it's not going to cause major disruption to your work unless you are working on some critical and urgent matter. Take a two to three-minute break, eat a banana or a handful of chana. If possible, carry chikki or a packet of chana to the meeting and care to share with stakeholders. Today you will share, in the next meeting, probably they will share. Why not make everybody around you healthy? Create that culture ☺.

Fourth Meal: Lunch

It is a meal to be eaten in the middle of the day and gives us the energy to manage our activities for the rest of the day. Ideally, it is to be lighter than our breakfast and heavier than the remaining meals. Adding curd/buttermilk to this meal gives us probiotics and aids the digestion process.

A good time to have it is within 90 minutes of your mid-meal or 4 hours after your breakfast and the options are:

Take anyone + Green Salad + Curd/Buttermilk.

- 1 chapatis/2 phulkas with veggies/chicken/fish + dal

- Steamed/sautéed vegetables with minimal spices.

- Dal rice (1 cup steamed rice) + ghee + methkut / homemade chutney

- Dal khichdi with veggies

- Grilled paneer/chicken/fish

- Multigrain paneer/chicken sandwich

- Any subway with just salt, pepper, and minimal sauces

- Sautéed mushroom/soya/chicken

- Panner/egg burjee + 1 chapati/2 slices of multigrain bread

Adding salads gives you good fibre and keeps you full. Avoid using any high-calorie dips along with it.

For most, lunch or dinner = Dal rice or chapati sabji, which is perfectly fine. Add ghee to your dal to enhance taste and get good fats too.

Mital: Did you say sandwich for lunch!

Mitali is a sales professional and is always on the move. She has been facing obesity issues and her irregular meals were the main reason behind it.

Me: Yes Mitali.

Mitali: But I have always eaten roti-sabji for lunch. If I eat a sandwich, I don't feel like I've had lunch.

Me: But you said you can't carry it, right?

Mitali: Yes, as I leave early from home, and the food is not ready.

Me: So, when and what do you eat?

Mitali: Generally, I skip lunch and have something once I reach the office around 4:00 p.m.

Me: That is the culprit. Your body craves food, so I am sure you overeat once you reach the office. To manage this hunger, you need to eat lunch and a multigrain or a brown bread sandwich is a good option.

Mitali: Still a sandwich!

Me: It's all psychological. From childhood, we've been eating a particular type of lunch as per our culture, so we always believe that's the best option. And I do not deny that. Even for me, the most satisfying lunch is home-cooked chapati/roti, dal – rice with a spoon of ghee and a portion of vegetables, served hot. But it's not always feasible due to work and other commitments, so whenever I am at home, I don't miss it.

Mitali: That's true

Me: You need to ensure that you give your body good food at the right time. Eating a sandwich will give you the required energy and help you manage food cravings.

Mitali: Sure, let me try it.

Me: See that you restrict the use of butter and sauces.

Mitali: I will do that.

If it were always possible for us to eat home-cooked food, then probably we would not be facing such rampant obesity issues. But there are practical challenges; hence I have specified a few other options which can be consumed for lunch.

But, if you always eat out, ensure that you eat from a good source and the usage of oil, spices, and sauces is minimal.

Thoda tari aur dalo, spicy nahi lag raha hai (Add more spice) …… You should not be doing this often.

Fifth Meal: Snack

4 baje ki chai and chai ke sath pakora, majjani life! (What else do you need, if you can have tea and fritters for a 4:00 p.m. meal)

No more if you have it daily ☺.

Let's talk about the most junk prone meal of the day: Snack.

The timing for this meal is normally in the late afternoon or early evening and it assumes a lot of importance. This is because it is the time of day when more than three-fourth of the working day is done, and we are slightly relaxed. Besides, during this time, most office canteens serve chats, pakoras (fritters), etc which are tempting. You may fall for it if you do not plan this meal well. Just like how the mid-meal ensures you have a light lunch, this meal will help you have a light dinner.

What are the options for this meal?

Take any one:

- Rajgiri/Groundnut/Til/Coconut chikki
- Makahana – 1 bowl
- Sprouts bhel
- Dry bhel
- Green salad
- Fruit
- Soya Chunks

- Chana Chat

- Sautéed Tofu

- Protein bars

- Homemade chivda

- Khakra

- Corn chat

This meal can be had in as little as five minutes, just like your mid-meal, so all that I mentioned for it applies to this meal too. If you still want to have your chai, then have it along with this meal. It will help to have it with minimum or no added sugar though.

Some may say that they reach home by 6:00 p.m., so do they really need this meal?

Absolutely, you need it. In my experience, whenever I have missed this meal, my urge to have chai and biscuits goes upon reaching home. Eat something, even if it's just two pieces of chikki is fine.

Let's now go to the last solid meal of the day – Dinner.

What's the first thing that comes to your mind, when I say dinner?

Post 9:00 p.m.

With family

TV time

A lot of food

What if I say, this meal must be finished before sunset or max by 7:30 p.m.

A few may raise their eyebrows!

I spoke to Shakti, a project manager with a big IT organisation. She starts her day early, but her workload doesn't allow her to reach home in time, due to which she has been eating late dinners. Also, she doesn't have a cook, so she has to cook her meals too.

Me: You need to have an early dinner.

Shakti: What did you say, 7:30 p.m. That is not possible. I reach home only by 8:30 p.m., then I start making dinner. So, it's only by 10, I can have dinner.

Me: Do you get dosa/uttapa/paratha in your canteen?

Shakti: Yes, it's available.

Me: So, have that for dinner.

Shakti: Dosa for dinner!

Me: Why not? It is food, it will give you energy. Just tell the cook, not to add butter. I am sure, you must be eating something when you reach home.

Shakti: Ya, I am hungry, so I mostly have tea and biscuits.

Me: See, that's the problem! Start having dosa or something healthy and filling around 7:00 p.m., then you will not need chai-biscuits.

Shakti: In fact, our canteen has more options; I can try that too.

Me: Yes, you should.

Shakti: So, are you saying that I should skip dinner, once I am home?

Me: You aren't skipping it, you are 7:00 p.m. meal is your dinner.

Eyebrows raised again, but with a smile.

Shakti: I got it.

Me: Let me know how it feels, maybe in a week.

I received her call exactly after a week.

Shakti: It's working fine, I am not getting hunger pangs anymore. But I don't get time with my family, as earlier we all sat together at the dinner table. In fact, that was the only time we all bonded together.

Me: Once you all get home, why don't you sit and talk, or play a game of cards, or watch your saas-bahu programme together? You don't need food to bond, right ☺.

Shakti: And another problem is that if I have dinner at 7:00 p.m., then I feel hungry around 9–9:30 p.m. and I cannot sleep on an empty stomach.

Me: You need not sleep on an empty stomach. Have a glass of milk around 9:00 p.m., get the required energy, and hit the bed before 10:30 p.m. In fact, having warm milk with added turmeric will not only help you be full but will induce sleep too. (No more sleepless nights)

And, if you don't like plain milk, you can add something (just ensure that it is not sugar)

Shakti: I think this will work.

Dinner is where most go wrong in terms of timings and portion. But making this one change will influence your health and fitness to a great extent. This gives enough time to your body to digest your food, unlike late dinners, where you immediately hit the bed. And undigested food is one of the main causes of acidity and bloating.

Dinner options: Same as suggested for lunch, but a smaller portion, have variations as required. Do not have the same foods for lunch and dinner to avoid boredom. Please note, this must be the last solid meal of the day.

We are done with the meal planning, let's summarise.

-**First Meal**: Water + dry fruits (4–5 soaked black raisins + 2 almonds)

To be taken within 15 mins of waking up.

-**Second Meal**: Breakfast

To be taken within 60 minutes of waking up.

-**Third Meal**: Mid-Meal

To be taken within 90–120 minutes post breakfast.

-**Fourth Meal**: Lunch

To be taken within 4 hours post breakfast.

-**Fifth Meal**: Snack

To be taken within 2–3 hours post-lunch

-**Sixth Meal**: Dinner

To be taken before 7:00 p.m. (max 7:30 p.m.)

-**Post-Dinner meal**

To be taken 1 hour before sleeping.

If you practice this for two to three weeks:

- Your food cravings will be reduced.

- You will not overeat.

- You will feel energetic.

- Your digestion will improve.

- You will get good sleep and enjoy amazing mornings.

Let's get going.

Chapter 9
Do You Have Cheat Meals?

Aasavari is a housewife, an ardent foodie and an old friend. I was discussing with her how one can stay healthy and still enjoy their meals.

Aasavari: Kya yehi khana hai pura life? Matlab pizza, pakoda, wada pav, cake, cookies ko dekhna bhi nahi hai? (Do I need to eat all of this throughout my life, what about pizzas, cookies, etc, Can I never have them?)

Me: What is your favourite food?

Aasavari: Wada pav (Indian burger).

Me: What if I tell you that you can have wada pav and still stay fit.

Aasavari: Yeh khake hi itna weight badh gaya hai, if I eat more, how will I lose weight? (I have gained weight eating all of these foods.)

Me: You will.

Aasavari: But wada pav has a lot of calories. I will eat it after I am back to 55 kgs.

Me: Don't worry about calories, just focus on eating five to six meals as suggested and have a cheat meal once a week.

Aasavari: Cheat meals?

Me: Yes, you heard it right. Let me explain. We are normal people and not professional athletes. They have a completely different mindset, different goals, and can stay aligned with stringent training and eating patterns for a long time. Plus, if you are a foodie like me, then you just can't stay away from tasty food. We get cravings and we try to delay them, thinking once we drop those extra kgs, we will indulge. What we call "Maan – Marna" (half-heartedly) is what we do, I told her.

Aasavari: That's true.

Me: Let's not do it. Like the way we say, "Hum ek baar jeete hai, ek baar marte hai, shaadi bhi ek baar hoti hai… aur pyar ek baar hi hota hai", let's extend the same to our taste buds. (We live only once, so let's live to the fullest.) Do you not want to have it and still stay aligned with your fitness goal?

Aasavari: Of course, I would love to have it and still get fit. Who would say no?

Then, let's talk about cheat meal. It's a meal where you allow yourself to consume any foods you want, without guilt. Yes, you can have what you want; once a week or once in 15 days.

Why Cheat Meal?

- To manage your cravings *(if you keep having them)*

- To reward yourself for a disciplined week *(self-motivation)*

- To make your journey exciting.

How to Plan?

- Decide the day you want to have it.

- Have it without any guilt and feel good.

- Now, this is an important step where most go wrong: Get back to your next planned meal. Just because you had a cheat meal, it doesn't permit you to skip your next meal (unless you are full). Also, remember it is a cheat meal and not a cheat day.

Let's say you choose Saturday afternoon to have the pizza of your choice. You got it delivered by your favourite restaurant and enjoyed every bite of it. It made you feel good and happy. What next? After some time, you may start feeling guilty. *(Why did I eat it, my weight will go up and so on...)* Guilt can be demotivating and may upset your mood. So, tell yourself that the cheat meal is done, and YOU NEED TO JUST GET BACK TO YOUR NEXT PLANNED MEAL, just like any other day. It is better to plan that next meal in advance, so you have no excuse to miss it.

Cheat meals give you a sense of satisfaction and motivate you to follow your planned meals in anticipation of your next cheat meal. It's also an opportunity to connect with your friends or families over lunch or social events.

A Few Guidelines

- Restrict it to **1 meal per week**, once in 2 weeks is even better.

- Stay away from aerated drinks to **avoid the sugar rush.**

- Limit/avoid **consumption of alcohol** *(When you take alcohol, you lose count of the pakoras/chicken lollypops you eat.)*

- Focus on **portion**. If you are done with 1 pizza, you need not order the next one.

- Eat with the **intent of enjoying your meal** and not with finishing and ordering more.

- Eat your **next meal as per the plan**. In fact, eat your pre-meal also, so you will not hog.

- Remember it is a cheat meal and **not cheat day** *(one meal in a day and not all meals)*.

- And lastly, tell yourself that you have been putting a lot of effort into your fitness and this is a **motivation for you** to focus better.

Chapter 10
Managing Social Events

Saal me ek baar hi birthday aata hai, ek party to banti hai (Birthdays come once a year, so it makes sense to celebrate it).

It's my project success party, I must go.

Its Diwali gala dinner, I cannot miss it.

It's my brother's engagement party, I need to be there.

It is a Friday night, come on, let's celebrate.

How many of you have felt like going to social events, but you didn't, thinking about weight gain? Because of this, how many of you have given some lame excuses to your friends?

I am sure there are many. That night, you would have sat at home missing the party and thinking about it the whole time and then cursing yourself for not going!

Let me tell you, you do not need to do that. Like we saw in the cheat meal discussion, it is fine to indulge in the foods of your choice once in a while. Treat these events as your cheat meal and enjoy them. Now, do not immediately call up your friends and plan a party. There are some guidelines to follow when you go for social dining. Let us look at them:

Have these thoughts ever come to your mind, while going to your favourite buffet restaurant?

I paid for it, so I'm going to Vasool it. (I have paid for it, so will extract a full value)

Aaj pura vasool karna hai (I am going to extract a full value)

Last time, ek desert choot gaya tha, aaj sab khana hai (Last time, I had missed out on the dessert, this time I will have everything.)

Aaaj pura din upvas karunga, aur phir tuth padonga (Will fast for the entire day and eat like nobody is watching.)

Let me tell you these thoughts are dangerous. Tumhare fitness journey ke liye Hanikarak hai! *(These thoughts are dangerous for your fitness journey)*

What is the point in pasia vasoling and then spending more money on dietician fees and acidity tablets? So, tell yourself that you are going to an event not just for the food, but also to connect with the host and other guests. When you do that, you shift your focus from food and the paisa-vasool attitude. Once you have managed this, then the next steps are not that difficult. Let's look at them too.

Tip: Always eat a light meal and go:

Most parties are late evenings, where food is served post 8:00 p.m., whereas you are used to finishing your dinner early. So, what happens is that by the time you get there, and you have not eaten anything, you would be super hungry. When we are hungry and there is a lot of food options in front of us, we might eat mindlessly. We might enjoy it at that moment, but later we may feel bad about it. Hence, eating a light meal or your planned meal before leaving for such events always helps.

But I am going to a dinner party, so if I eat and go, I will not feel like eating there, some of you might say this. *You are right, but you would also want to stick to your healthy eating habits which you have picked up and would not want to feel guilty post eating.*

I suggest you eat something light (like a snack) rather than going on an empty stomach, so you can still enjoy the party, minus the guilt.

Tip: Remember the Portion-Control rule, even when you dine out:

Eating smaller portions allows you to eat your favourite food while keeping calories in check. It ensures that you do not unnecessarily hog. If you are going to a buffet or a la carte, you will have the option of 2-course, 3-course or even 4-course meals, what we typically call soups, starters, main course, and deserts. The first thing is you need not have all four meals. I know you have paid for it, but by now you are already out of the Paisa-vasool attitude.

- You can always take soups and starters and avoid the other two.

- Or you can take starters and deserts and avoid the main course completely.

- Some people eat only soups and starters, which is also fine.

And if you are the one who wants to eat all 4, this may help you follow portion control:

Take your serving plate and fill 50% of it with a few starters. Prefer grilled/tandoor over fried ones. So, if there is the option of panner/chicken tikka, prefer it over paneer pakora or chicken lollipop. I know the fried foods are tempting; if you still want to have them, restrict them to one piece.

By now half your plate is full. Now, fill another 1/4th portion with salads. There is generally a good spread right from plain salads like cut cucumber, carrot, etc. to the ones covered in some *(yummy looking)* dressings. If it is mayo-based, then avoid it as it has oil and sugar. If you want to make your salad moist, look for lime or vinegar-based dips. There is also a mixed salad, which will have sprouts added to it, you can take that too.

You still have 1/4th plate empty, and you should fill it with the right food. The reason is that when we see space, our mind gets tricked into adding something and then we may end up adding whatever is available. Add a tandoori roti or a paratha. You may be surprised with roti and starter combination, as roti is considered a part of my main course. Recollect what we mentioned earlier, having carbs along with proteins enhances their value. Also, it keeps you full. Most starters are protein-rich and adding a position of bread will serve the purpose. Now your plate is full, and you should focus on enjoying your meal.

We are not done yet! There is an option of soup or a beverage as sides. Prefer a clear or thin soup over those thick soups. If you like beverages (most of them are complementary), then avoid the aerated ones and have lime or jaljira based with no or minimal added sugar.

Now some self-control: once you finish the plate, you should not go for a second helping, if you plan to have mains and desserts too. If you are not planning to have them, then a repeat of starters is fine, but this time take only 20–30% of what you had taken earlier.

Let's go to the main course. In a typical buffet, there is a huge spread for mains, right from three to four varieties of rice, noodles, pasta, a few rich curries, dals, papads, chutneys, etc. Opt for a medium-size plate and add a small portion of rice with one or two portions of non-rich curries. Avoid papads if possible. Eat slowly and once you are done, do not take a second serving. You can finish your meal here and avoid desserts. But there is a huge spread of lip-smacking desserts and saying no can be difficult.

Indulging in deserts. You will have a tough time choosing, as the spread is huge. Here, the best thing is to have a smaller plate and take a minimum portion. Also, once you are done serving yourself, go back to your table, sit, and eat. I have seen many standing near the dessert counter and eating and immediately refilling the plate. Enjoy your dessert and once you are done, clear the plate. Never repeat the desert.

a. Alcohol – If you indulge in drinking alcohol, restrict it to not more than one serving.

Tip: Few more things to look at:

a. *Ek roti khalo, muzhe company milegi aur khana bhi waste nahi hoga, said Adhiraj to his friend Kapil. (Have one more bread to give me company).*

No yaar, I am full, replied Kapil.

Arre 1 se kya hoga, adhiraj added further as he instructed the attendant to serve. (Eating just 1 more will not make you fat).

And that's how Kapil had one more roti and curry (He *had finished his plate earlier but had not requested the attendant to clear it.)*

Have the attendant remove your plate as soon as you are finished. If you keep the plate in front of you once you are done, there are chances you may eat again just to give company to your friend, colleague, family member or to finish the unfinished portions.

It is our moral responsibility to not waste food, but that doesn't mean eating more than what you need. Be more responsible when the food is served. If you cannot finish the portions, get them packed and give them to the needy, you will get a blessing too. Nowadays restaurants are tied up with NGOs to serve food to the needy.

In good restaurants, you can also check with the chef regarding the ingredients of your meal and I have seen chefs enjoy talking about it too. So, check how your food is made, suggest if you do not want a particular ingredient.

b. One last thing, chew your food properly and this will help the digestion process.

Tip: Plan your food itinerary in advance.

How?

Thanks to our smartphones, we can access the food menu online. Decide your choices based on your goals and order like a pro. This will help you in eating the right meal.

If you follow these basic guidelines, you can enjoy social events occasionally without any guilt. (Fortnightly or monthly)

Chapter 11
How Good Is Your Digestion?

Nakul works as a sales executive in a manufacturing firm. He has been suffering from acidity issues for the past few months. We discussed how it could be resolved.

Nakul: My mornings are really bad. Half the time I feel acidic or bloated, and it spoils my first half of the day. Can you help?

Me: This has become a common problem across the globe and is increasing day by day. It is not just because of the food we eat, but also how and when we eat.

Nakul: But I normally eat home-cooked food and I carry it to the office even.

Me: Is it? What time do you have lunch?

Nakul: That depends on work, but I try finishing it between 1:30 and 2:00 p.m.

Me: And how much time does it take you to finish lunch?

Nakul: I don't eat much, just two chapatis and veggies, so I finish it in less than five minutes, so I can take a long walk to digest my food. (As if his boss is giving him a prize for finishing lunch in record time, so he can work more!)

Me: That is the problem Nakul. Have you heard people say, "Chew your food 32 times."

Nakul: Ya, but what has that got to do with my problem?

Me: You tend to go for a walk to digest your food, but you are not following the first step for digestion.

Nakul: What is that?

Me: Our digestion starts in the mouth. (I pointed to an image of a digestive track on my laptop.) If the food is chewed properly (32 times), saliva glands are activated to secret saliva. Saliva moistens the throats and aids digestion. So, if you don't chew properly, you miss this step for good digestion. If you finish your food in five minutes, you know that you are not chewing your food well. If time is a constraint, then you can shorten your walk.

Nakul: I can do that, how much time should I spare?

Me: It's not about allocating time as such. Instead, focus on your food, appreciate the flavours, enjoy the taste and you will be able to do it right. On average it takes 15–20 minutes to finish your lunch/dinner.

Nakul: Sure, I will do that.

Me: Try it for two weeks and get back to me. It's not going to be easy, as you are not used to it, but gradually you will be able to do it.

I got his call in the next nine days.

Nakul: My acidity problem has reduced. Thanks for your advice.

Me: So how much time does it take to have lunch?

Nakul: Twenty minutes…

Me: Great, follow this rule when eating all your meals and you will see further benefits. And what about your post-lunch walks? *(I thought he would have stopped walking due to lack of time.)*

Nakul: I am still doing it. *(If you decide, you can definitely find the time ☺.)*

Making a simple change like chewing properly can do wonders for your digestive health.

When you eat, your digestive system works objectively, so your body can absorb the nutrients and use them for energy and growth. If this system does not work well, then even if you consume the best quality foods, it will not get absorbed in your body, and won't do any good.

When you take a bite, your teeth start breaking it down. This is where the fun lies. If you **chew properly (32 times),** there are two benefits:

- You break the food, making it easy to pass down.

- Salivary glands are activated to secrete adequate saliva, which helps in initiating the digestion process.

From there, the semi-digested food enters the oesophagus and from there to the stomach, where the digestion process continues. If food is not chewed properly, it puts additional pressure on the stomach and impacts the digestion process. Glands in your stomach lining make stomach acids and enzymes that help in breaking down food. Muscles of your stomach play a role in terms of mixing the food with these digestive juices.

When the digestion process is impacted, the stomach throws this acid out (*reflux*) and that is the reason you sometimes get the acidic taste in your mouth. (*It is an indication of poor digestion.*) From the stomach, the semi-digested food is then passed on to the small intestine where it is further digested and absorbed.

There are finger-like structures present in the small intestine called villi which play a major role in the absorption of nutrients in your bloodstream. If this doesn't function well, then your body is not able to absorb and make use of the food you eat.

When someone says, "*Kitna bhi aacha kaho, mere body ko kuch fayda hi nahi hota,*" it is due to inadequate functionality of the villi. (*Even though I eat good food, it doesn't help my body.*)

And regular consumption of junk food slows down the villi! Hence, eat the right food, not just for fat loss, but also to enable the absorption of nutrients.

Food is passed to the large intestine, where the digestion process is completed, and the waste is thrown out of the body. This sums up the digestion process and it takes around four to five hours depending on the type of food consumed.

Undigested food causes acidity and that is why it is advised to finish your last meal of the day at least four hours before you sleep. If you sleep immediately after you eat or if you consume heavy dinners, you may experience acidity or reflux the next morning, because you didn't give your body enough time to digest the food. This impacts your sleep as well. With undigested food in the stomach, your body is focused on supplying more blood to your stomach than your brain to get sound sleep.

A bad digestive system is the root cause of so many issues.

I discussed with Venu, a professor, about his constipation problem.

Venu: I spend at last 45 minutes in the washroom every single day and then I feel heavy the entire day and don't feel like eating much.

Me: What do you have for breakfast?

Venu: Since I don't feel hungry, I take fruit juice with no sugar.

Me: Why don't you eat some fruit instead?

Venu: Oh, I don't like fruits, but I drink fruit juice on daily basis.

Me: What do you eat for lunch/dinner?

Venu: It's mostly dal khichdi or some preparation of rice.

Me: Don't you eat vegetables?

Venu: I only eat panner and potatoes.

Me: What about pulses and greens?

Venu: I feel heavy, so I avoid pulses particularly.

Me: You need to start adding fibre to your meals, this will help solve your problem. You are suffering from constipation and eating fibre-rich foods will help you ease it.

Venu: How?

Me: Eat fibre-rich foods and drink enough water.

What is Constipation?

We saw that as a part of the digestion process, waste products are eliminated by the large intestine. Now, imagine, if this waste is not flushed out for days, the kind of environment it will create in your body. You can compare it to a choked sink, with food particles and other waste accumulating and stinking up the place. It's the same with our body when constipated.

For food to move through the long-coiled digestive track, it needs optimum pressure. When that pressure is not available, the food moves slowly through the track and it becomes difficult to throw it out of our body.

For instance, take a set of rolled papers and try passing them through a long-coiled tube of approximately 30 feet. You'd need someone to push it to take it out, right? The same is the case with our body, we need a push (pressure) to eliminate the waste. Enter the hero, **fibre,** in the scene. Fibre provides the required push and helps relieve you of constipation. It acts like a utensils scrubber and collects the waste from the body and helps push it out. Whole grains, fruits, and vegetables are good sources of fibre.

Fibre also plays a role in keeping you full and beating your hunger pangs. Hence, you feel full for a long time when you eat a whole apple compared to drinking apple juice.

So, adding fruits, vegetables, and whole-grain chapatis/rotis to your meals will give you relief from constipation.

Venu: But I take fruit juice every day, some days I even drink two glasses of juice.

Me: I mentioned fruit (whole fruit) and not fruit juice. When a fruit is juiced, you get the taste, but lose the fibre.

Venu: Ahhh… I have been buying premium quality juices for the past two years now.

Me: Instead, eat some fruit, you will get the much-needed fibre and you also save a good amount of cash.

Venu: Sure, I will do that.

Me: Similarly, add a portion of veggies to your meals.

Venu: Will this solve my problem?

Me: There is one more thing to look at.

Venu: What's that?

Me: You need to start drinking …a lot of water as it helps in relieving constipation.

Venu: How much water is needed?

Me: For every 20 kgs of your ideal weight, you need one litre of water. If your ideal weight is 60 kgs, you need three litres every day. Over and above this, whenever you feel thirsty or you experience dryness in your throat, you should drink water. I had shown you earlier how to calculate ideal body weight (Weight in centimetres – 100). So, calculate your ideal weight and start consuming the required water.

Venu: But 3.5 litres is too much, I drink a maximum of three to four glasses every day, how do I take more?

Me: Try this:

- Keep a one-litre water bottle handy at your desk and fill it when you start your day. Put a 30-minute reminder on your mobile.

- Every time it beeps, drink water (sometimes a sip or even more, depending on how thirsty you are).

- Make a note about how many bottles are done.

- You just need to finish 3–3.5 bottles in a day.

Venu: Sure, I will start this tomorrow.

Me: You may find it difficult on day 1, but over a period, you will reach your quota.

Venu: Thanks

Water

Water is a universal solvent, and our body consists of 70–80% of water said the teacher to all her students.

So how much should we drink, asked one of the students?

Ensure that you do not take a filled water bottle home, replied the teacher.

Ok ma'am, as he emptied the bottle and the class cheered.

How many of you have heard this in school?

Still, if you have any questions, why does the body need water?

Jinda rehne ke liye (to live)!

There are ways to make this superfluid work best for us:

- Drink more water in the first half of the day and reduce the quantity gradually post-sunset. This will help you get the required quota and will not disturb your sleep due to a restroom visit.

- Also, never gulp the water, drink it slowly, allowing the saliva to mix with water. You are drinking a super fuel that does wonders to your body, so sit, relax, and sip it calmly.

- Avoid drinking too much water immediately before and after meals.

- Other than drinking water, you can also consume fruits like watermelon which contains a lot of water. Similarly, consuming certain water-rich vegetables will help further.

Constipation, acidity, bloating and reflux are conditions that are linked to a bad lifestyle and cause havoc. But they can be prevented by making simple changes to the way you live.

There are various causes of acidity, but the ones which I want to highlight are:

- Skipping breakfast

- Keeping long gaps between meals

- Late dinners (*not giving time for digestion*)

- Eating a lot of spicy food

- Low consumption of fibre

- Multiple cups of tea and coffee

- Lack of sleep

Time and again, all these habits point to an unhealthy lifestyle, and the way we are progressing through this book, I am sure we will be able to tackle it as we reach the finish line. Mindful eating, drinking enough water, consuming fibre-rich foods and exercising regularly helps keep these digestion related issues at bay. We are gradually inching towards holistic fitness.

Chapter 12
Let's Shop the Right Way

Adil works as a sales manager in an insurance firm. He plays cricket with his colleagues every Sunday.

Adil: We are going to buy groceries this Sunday, I cannot come to the cricket match.

Rajiv (colleague): You can do your shopping in the morning and come back, we have booked the turf for the 11:00 a.m. slot.

Adil: We are going to the mall; it will take the entire day.

Rajiv: One full day just to buy groceries!

Adil: We will leave home around 10:00 a.m. On reaching the mall, we will go to the kids' zone first, where Aditi and Ahan will spend at least one hour. Then, we will go to the food mart to get the groceries, from there to the food court for lunch, followed by a movie at 2:00 p.m. and if the kids are hungry, then some snack and coffee around 6:00 p.m. So, by the time, we reach home, it will be 7:00 p.m.

Rajiv: So, you are actually going for a movie and lunch and you plan to buy groceries too!

Adil: No, that's how we buy groceries and veggies for the entire week. Who gets time during weekdays? Plus, we get all the stuff in one place and even the kids enjoy themselves. So, it becomes a family outing.

Rajiv: Sure Adil, have a great time, we will see you on Monday at work.

Adil: You too have a great match; I will be there for the next one.

Is this har ghar ki kahani? *(Does every household have the same story?)*

How many can relate to this?

This is how grocery shopping has changed over the last decade, so I thought of adding this topic to make your shopping a memorable experience.

Before we get there, let's have a look at the **current food scenario.**

Food adulteration and food handling malpractices have gone up.

Premature plucking of fruits and vegetables is one of them. This is carried out to increase their shelf life and avoid early ripening.

These fruits and vegetables are not grown near our homes, but in farmlands far away from city limits. These are then put in trucks and transported to a distributor or a whole seller and from there to the stores and then to our homes. This whole cycle takes 2–3 days or even more.

Hence to prevent their damage (overripe), they are plucked before they reach the actual plucking time.

This looks good from the business point of view but think about the impact on the quality of the product. Fruits and vegetables get nutrition from the soil through stems. When they are plucked before time, they do not get the complete nutrition and when we consume them, we too do not get complete nutrition. The apple which you buy from a supermarket may still look bright red and fresh from the outside, but it lacks the nutrients within.

So, should we not eat them?

We should, but buy it from a good source. Rather than buying it from malls that stock them for long, buy it from local vendors or the farmer's market. They sell a limited stock, but it's fresh. In fact, some of them are farmers who pluck them the same morning or perhaps the previous day and they do not stock it for long, so the quality is not degraded. For ages, we have been doing this before the mall culture hit us and changed our habits. In addition to this, the use of **fertilisers and pesticides** has gone up, which further impacts our health. We cannot do much about it but we can certainly buy from the right source.

During the COVID-19 pandemic, when the malls and supermarkets were closed, these small vendors came to our rescue.

Every other day, we read about **milk adulteration.** We also see videos about colours that are added to vegetables, wax applied to fruits, etc., to make them look fresh. **Cows are injected with hormones** so they can give more milk, and chickens are given **growth hormones**, so we get more flesh. All these bad practices are rampant. When we eat such food, these chemicals and hormones also reach our body. This is the reason so many kids reach puberty at an earlier age. **PCOD and PCOS** cases are growing at a rapid rate.

Have you seen how food is transported?

We know it is done through trucks, but a closer look will reveal that the same truck is used to transport both vegetables and livestock. Trucks are overloaded and people sit on top of the loads, so imagine the pressure it puts on the produce beneath. I am not saying this happens everywhere, but I've seen such practices happening, and we as consumers are unaware of it.

Have you ever been to sabji mandi *(the wholesale market for fruits and vegetables)?*

If you want first-hand experience with food handling, then you should. You will see the vegetables and fruits lying on the floor. Small vendors bargain, stamp and sometimes even crush your exotic broccoli and zucchini. And we buy the same produce when it reaches the store at an exclusive price. We eat it with pride thinking about the great nutrition we are consuming.

These are some examples and there are many more that impact the nutritional value of our food.

"Food is for hunger; Nutrition is for the body."

If you understand this statement, half the game is won. So, the next time you see a potato, do not think about French fries.

Now let us go back and plan food shopping the right way.

Tip: Make a shopping list: Sounds boring, but it works well in terms of not buying unnecessary things.

"Dada, look at this new flavour of mayo, let's try this."

"Wow, there is an offer of buy two get two free in my favourite cookies, let's buy one more."

"This pack of cookies is on discount for the first time, let's buy at least two."

These conversations are common.

When you don't have a list in hand, you may end up buying all these offers. If you have the list, you will think twice. Making a list takes a few minutes; ensure that it is made taking inputs from everyone at home.

A good shopping list saves time and money + unwanted calories.

Tip: Have a meal before you step out: Never go on an empty stomach, especially to a food store.

There are several options and if have not eaten, there are chances you may feel hungry just by looking at the display of food. Add to it the long cash counter queues and the way food items are placed strategically near the cash counter. It's difficult to control the craving and then you may end up buying unnecessary items. Recall your last few shopping encounters and ask yourself, did you buy a few unwanted items while standing in a queue? If yes, then this tip will help you.

If you get into the practice of having a meal before you shop, then you may not have cravings; you may just look at those items as you pass through the queue and may not buy anything. When we are hungry, we see food everywhere and then we tend to buy more food items. So, eating and going will save you a lot of money + unwanted calories.

Tip: Take a small shopping cart – We try to fill empty spaces; may it be your lunch plate or your wardrobe or even your shopping cart. Hence take a small one, so it will get full quicker.

Ideally, opt for a shopping basket, rather than a small cart, if your list is small.

The benefits of taking a shopping basket are two-fold:

- It will fit limited products

  Since you need to carry the basket unlike a cart, you will not overload it and will finish your shopping quicker. It saves time and money.

Tip: Do not take kids shopping – Have you seen kids sitting in a shopping cart and parents pushing it across the shopping mall?

Keeping kids engaged for long is a task. Also, there are a lot of kid-related products like chocolates, biscuits, jams, etc placed on the shelves and smart marketing campaigns are run to attract their attention. Parents are compelled to get these unhealthy foods, not just to keep the kids happy, but also for their peace of mind. Not all products are healthy, and we must realise that kids' obesity is growing at an alarming rate and this unplanned shopping is just adding to it. Hence avoid taking kids.

Do not make shopping look like a family outing by taking everyone along. This will help you save time, money + unwanted calories.

Tip: Avoid sampling counters:

Sir, would you like to taste these baked cookies, it's a new product launched yesterday. It is low in calories and has no added sugar, said a salesgirl to Parag as he manoeuvred his trolley through the mall.

"Yes," he said, as he extended his hand to take a piece.

"How is it sir," asked the girl with a smile?

"It is good," replied Parag with an accent.

"We have 30% off on this, would you like to buy one packet?"

"Ya, I liked it." (How can Parag say no?)

And an item got added to his shopping cart… *(which was not on his list)*

There are a lot of sampling counters, especially on weekends. And, if your cart looks full, there are high chances that the counter salesperson will approach you upfront. *(This is another benefit of taking a basket or a small cart.)*

Also, our chances of tasting an item go up if we are hungry (This is another benefit of having a meal prior.)

What happens post tasting is that they will ask for your feedback (which is right) and you may give a positive one. Then, they talk about irresistible offers.

Sir, it's buy one get one free, only for today.

Then you assume your moral responsibility to try (buy) the product. Hence, staying away from these counters will save money and unwanted calories.

Tip: Be smart about offers: We often see these banners, especially at the start of the month or during festivals:

Buy 3, get 2 free.

Offer only for today.

This product is on offer for the first time.

49-99-199-499… (1 less than round figure)

Big Sale

Seeing such attractions, we rush to those counters to buy them. I am not saying we should say no to every such offer. Decide based on your need and not the offer. Recall your last shopping visit and check your kitchen cabinet. There are high chances you may find an item you bought on offer and is still lying their unused. Sometimes what happens is, since you've already bought it, you consume it *(adding to unwanted calories at times)*. Just be smart and vigilant about your purchases and it will help you a lot.

These are some of the tried and tested tricks. Start implementing them and you will go light on your wallet and stomach too. There are multiple products, and we are literally spoilt for options when we go shopping.

Let's look at the next chapter to understand how to pick a particular product that will help us stay aligned with our fitness journey.

Chapter 13

Read the Label

Simmi and her brother Vishal had gone to a mall to buy their monthly groceries.

Simmi: Wow, this is what I was looking for! (She had picked up a packet of low sugar cookies from the shelf of a supermarket.) These are low in sugar, I can eat them without guilt.

Vishal: Check the ingredients Simmi.

Simmi: It is clearly written no sugar, what else to check for?

Vishal: (He turned the product over and read the label.) It has 8 grams of trans fat.

Simmi: So much!

Vishal: Yes, hence it is necessary to read the nutrition labels before buying a product. This will help you make informed choices.

Simmi: Thanks… (She kept the cookies back on the rack and continued with her shopping.)

Eating habits have changed over a decade. With supermarkets and malls coming up in every nook and corner, consumers are spoilt for choice. Further, in each product, there are multiple brands to choose from. Also, a lot of sugar-free, fat-free, baked, low salt products have been introduced to lure health-conscious consumers. Not all these products are healthy, even though they are branded as **health products.** Consumers also tend to buy a lot of off-the-shelf products from a convenience point, but some of them may be harmful to their health.

Additionally, higher disposable income and social media have influenced our shopping patterns. Hence, it is important to read nutrition labels to make the right choices.

Mostly, all packaged foods have a nutrition label, which provides the information necessary to know what we are eating, and it also serves as a base to compare similar products. Some consumers are allergic to certain ingredients and reading a label will help in avoiding such products. This chapter intends to help you read the label and is not about branding any product good or bad. That I leave to you once you read the label.

Let's read a Nutrition Label:

It has multiple things to look at, let's go through it one by one. Let me tell you that not all products will capture every piece of information listed below.

Serving Size: This is the amount of food that is typically eaten at one time. It can be in terms of pieces, weight, cups, etc.

Servings per container: It specifies the number of servings per package/box/container. In the example below, the package has 2 servings.

So, if you eat the entire package in one meal, you are eating a larger portion which can lead to weight gain.

It is recommended to eat from the plate and not the package to avoid eating more servings.

Nutrition Facts	
Serving Size 1 cup (200 gms)	
Servings per container 2	
Amount Per Serving	
Calories 240	Calories from Fat 110
	% Daily Value
Total Fat 12 g	18%
Saturated fat 3g	15%
Trans fat 3g	
Cholesterol 30mg	10%
Sodium 470mg	20%
Total Carbohydrates 31g	10%
Dietary Fiber 0g	0%
Sugars 5g	
Protein 5g	
Vitamin A	4%
Vitamin C	2%
Calcium	20%
Iron	4%

Nutrition Labels

Calories – It specifies the number of calories per serving (*not in the entire package*).

In this example, there are 240 calories in one serving. If you eat the entire package, which is 2 servings, you are consuming 480 calories (double).

Calories from fat – 110 calories are obtained from fat, which is almost 45%!

It signifies that it is a fat-rich food, and you may want to stay away from it.

Total fat – One serving will give you 12 grams of fat and has 3 grams of trans-fat.

% Daily Value – This helps to evaluate how a particular food fits into your daily nutrient intake. It compares how much of a nutrient is in one serving to how much of that nutrient you should consume in a day. The percentages are based on a daily diet of 2,000 calories.

If % DV is less than 5%, then it is on the lower side and if this is more than 20%, it is on the higher side. If you look at the above example, the % DV for fat is 18%, which means if you eat 1 serving, then you will cover 18% of your daily allowed fat limit.

The label also mentions other elements like carbs, protein, cholesterol, sodium, vitamins, and minerals and is to be interpreted in terms of % DV or the quantity mentioned (grams in the example).

Some labels will have information on **Added Sugars**. It refers to sugars that are added during the processing of foods. Foods high in added sugar are not recommended.

There are high chances that in a supermarket, you may not be able to read the entire label, so looking at a few critical parameters also help.

Bare minimum, look at calories from fat, sugar, trans-fat, % DV. It will allow you to make the right decision. Now that you know how to read a label, you can decide on which food products you should buy to suit your fitness goal.

In the next chapter, let's look at cooking the right way to gain maximum benefits.

Chapter 14
Do You Cook Right?

You have got the best ingredients from the right sources. You have also read the nutrition labels correctly. Now, let's cook the right way.

Archana and her daughter just got a few vegetables and fruits from a local market.

Archana: Sabji ko thik se clean karo, thoda soap bhi laga na. (Thoroughly clean the vegetables, apply some soap too.)

Daughter: Mummy yeh sabji hai, jo cook hone wali hai, koi fruit nahi, jo me direct khane wali hoo. (This vegetable will be cooked before eating, unlike fruit.)

Archana: Pata nahi, kaha kaha rakhi hogi (Not sure how it was handled).

Daughter: Thik hai, (Fine), as she continued the cleaning process.

How many of you actually do this or have done this?

I am not talking about COVID times, where we literally wash every item we get home.

Tip: Cleaning Vegetables and Fruits

We should clean them before consumption to get rid of germs since they pass through various hands before getting into our shopping basket. Washing will remove some of the germs and prevent them from entering our body. Especially root vegetables like onion, sweet potatoes, ginger, beetroots, radish, etc need to be cleaned thoroughly to remove soil and dirt. But some people resort to scrubbing them, the way we do our stained clothes, which is not needed. Over-washing can also remove some good elements which are present on the surface, and we might lose them.

Tip: Fine Chopping

For convenience, we tend to buy chopped vegetables and even fruits from the supermarket.

We are now aware of the time taken for a vegetable or fruit to reach the shelf of a supermarket from the time it is plucked. If we are going to get the chopped versions, imagine the nutrition loss. *(Do remember: Food is for hunger; Nutrition is for the body).*

The problem is not just compromised nutrition, it is how we assume that we are eating healthy food. And when we don't get desired results, we feel demotivated!

Cutting fruits or vegetables exposes them to oxygen and light, and sometimes heat, all of which affect the retention of vitamins in food. Also, in some fruits and vegetables, the nutrients are available in the outer layer, which gets lost in the process of heavy washing.

Hence, avoid buying pre-cut produce. If you cut it at home, do not store it long but consume it immediately. Whole fruit will keep longer than pre-cut fruit.

What is the right way to clean and cut?

- Wash your hands before washing fruits and vegetables.

- Clean your products well in running water, without using soap.

- Remove dirt and soil of root vegetables.

- Do not finely chop and preserve.

- If you must pre-cut for convenience, eat any pre-cut fruits in a day and any pre-cut vegetables in two days.

Tip: Spices

It was a Friday afternoon, Pushkar had just come back from college and was very hungry. He asked his mom for food and his mom made fresh food for him. *(Lucky are the ones who get hot food served by their moms.)*

After taking the first bite of aloo gobi sabji:

Pushkar: Yeh sabji kitni fiki hai, masala dala nahi kya? (This is so bland, have you not added spice?)

Mom: Masala jada nahi khana chaiyee. (One should not eat too much spice.)

Pushkar: Ha, per thoda spicy to hona hi chaiyee, nahi to kay maja, thoda masala dalo upper se. (Right, but there has to be some spice, can you add some now?)

Mom: Ye lo bottle and dalo jitna dalna hai, kal mat bolna acidity ho gayi, as she handed over the red chilli powder. (Take this bottle and add how much spice you want, but later, don't complain about acidity.)

Pushkar sprinkled the masala on his food and had a merry lunch.

Spices and masalas add rich flavour to our food without adding any calories. How can we miss the aroma of pav bhaji while passing by a fast-food corner? In fact, that is what drives us to eat it. And it's more than taste, what they bring to the table is important to note. Some spices like ginger and turmeric have anti-inflammatory properties, while others like cumin and cinnamon help with digestion.

But when we overdo anything, it will have side effects. Consumption of excess spices over a long period can damage the delicate membrane of the stomach, the food pipe and cause acidity and indigestion. There are ideal measurements available for the usage of each spice, but the rule of thumb says, add spice in a way that it will enhance the taste of your food and not supersede it. Eg., You are having grilled panner and want to add chat masala to make it tangy. Panner has good taste. So, when you add chat masala, ensure that the basic taste of panner is not compromised to make it tangy. If it does, then you have added too much spice.

Tip: Sauces

As such, you need to avoid them, but still, if you want to have it, add enough to moisten the food.

Aaryan, a seven-year-old kid had gone to Europe on vacation with his parents. He was excited to see the Eiffel Tower as he had read about the Wonders of the World in school. After waiting in a queue for 45 minutes and seeing the monument including the view from the North, he was on top of the world. But as he came down, he was tired and hungry. His mom took him to a nearby restaurant to have a quick meal and he ordered his favourite, French fries. Eating French fries in France was a part of his to-do list, so how could he miss it!

Aaryan: Where is my ketchup, he asked the cashier?

Cashier: Twenty cents more.

Aaryan: You do not offer it for free?

Cashier: Nope.

Aaryan looked at his mom asking for more money.

Mom: Do you really need it?

Aaryan: Ya, I cannot eat fries without ketchup.

His mom handed over the 20 cents and got the sachet of ketchup. Aaryan enjoyed his meal.

We are so used to having sauces that sometimes we cannot eat without them. Imagine you are eating a good multigrain sandwich with lots of veggies but dipped in mayo and ketchup. Think about the nutritional value of that meal. Sauces have a lot of sugar and other added preservatives which is of no use to the body.

There are so many sauces available, tomato-based, mayo-based, vinegar-based, etc. It is good to avoid the mayo-based completely and buy the others only after reading the nutrition label and use it sparingly.

Homemade chutneys can be a good replacement for sauces, and they taste very good.

I had been to one of the restaurants in North India, where they served this garlic-based chutney as a side. It was amazing, so I generally asked the attendant how it was made? To my surprise, he told me the recipe too.

Try it out: Take a cup of fresh curd, add a few pods of crushed garlic, and a pinch of salt and chat masala. It goes very well as a side.

Tip: Cookware and high flame

Sharvari was talking to her niece, Priya, about the use of oil and how it leads to weight gain and hence she avoids it, using her non-stick utensils.

Sharvari: I only use a non-stick pan to cook my meals, so I do not need much oil.

Priya: That is great, when did you get it?

Sharvari: My aunt gifted it to me when I got married. It has been more than 14 years and see, it's still the same.

Priya: Fourteen years! And you still use it? Is the coating still intact?

Sharvari: What is that?

Priya: Non-stick cookware usually has a coating over it, and it comes off over time.

Sharvari: How does it happen? I wash it properly every time I use it.

Priya: Non-stick utensils require extra care and handling as any sharp objects; metal spatulas can compromise the coating of these utensils. Using wooden or silicon cookware is an ideal option because such materials are less abrasive and do not cause damage to your cookware.

Sharvari: Oh, is it dangerous to use once the coating is off?

Priya: It is toxic and releases chemicals and it must not be used for cooking.

Sharvari: I will throw it away.

Priya: Absolutely!

We use the best possible ingredients and add good quality spices to make our food nutritious and tasty, but we do not pay much attention to the utensils that we cook in.

Cooking in utensils made of stainless steel, cast iron, glass and clay pots add extra health benefits. On the other hand, there are some materials like ceramic-coated, aluminium, Teflon-coated and damaged non-stick that may pose health threats if you cook food in them.

Traditionally, we have been using earthen cookware, and it is used even today in rural areas. No wonder people there are healthy.

In cities, lack of time and maintenance of such cookware, have pushed people to look at more convenient options like non-stick and aluminium.

But then, we miss out on the benefits of earthen cookware that includes their ability to absorb moisture due to their porous nature, letting heat circulate slowly through the food being cooked, making it aromatic, and retaining the nutrition.

Emotional Connect

Sometimes there are emotions attached to utensils, especially if they are gifted by loved ones during the marriage. So, you do not think about replacing them and use them for a lifetime.

I am not suggesting that you throw them away, instead, use them for some other work like gardening or some artwork and get the right ones for cooking.

Have a good look at your kitchen and replace the damaged utensils immediately. If possible, reintroduce earthen cookware (at least for weekends).

Tip: Cooking on a high flame

Jara gas ko tej kar, muzhe late ho raha hai, said Prita to her cook. (Please put the gas on high flame, I am getting late for work)

Ji madam, ho gaya ab, as she turned the knob. (Sure ma'am)

Everyone is in a rush today to catch the train, to reach the office, etc, but we need to give adequate time for our food to get cooked. Cooking on a high flame will get breakfast ready quickly, but the food will lose its nutrient value. There was a time when food used to get cooked in earthen pots on fire, which made the food tasty and nutritious. We cannot afford to do this now, but at least cook on low flame. When you do that, the nutrition is kept intact, and it also adds more flavour to the food.

Tip: Usage of Oils

Oil is an essential part of cooking and cannot be avoided. Proper usage of oil not just enhances the flavour but also ensures that the nutrients from the food get absorbed well in the body. Also, a plain khichadi doesn't taste as good as a khichadi with that tadka on top.

With a plethora of options available like coconut, sunflower, mustard, rice bran, olive oils how do we choose?

Use what is traditional and locally available to you. So, if you as a kid had had meals prepared in coconut oil, that suits you the best. Or if you are in North India, mustard oil will give you better benefits.

You will rarely see an obese kid in the coastal area who consumes coconut oil daily. However, when the same person migrates to other cities, often his health becomes poor or he suffers from obesity, mainly because of giving up on traditional food habits and opting for quick fixes and change in oil.

The food that you have been brought up on helps you thrive better.

Olive oil may suit people in colder climates. However, it does not give us any additional health benefits. Also, the heating point of each oil is different.

So, you definitely cannot fry pakoras in olive oil meant for salad dressing.

Apart from this, we have refined oils and cold-pressed oils.

Always prefer cold-pressed oil, as it is extracted by using optimum pressure and is not exposed to high temperatures, unlike commercial oils. Also, it keeps the nutrient value intact giving the desired health benefits.

In the case of commercially made oils, since they are exposed to a high temperature to extract all the oil possible, their nutrient value is often compromised. However, you may still get more oil at a lower price!

Consumption should be restricted to 500 ml per person for the month and cooking methods influence it too. E.g.: Some vegetables taste better with oil added on top rather than cooking in the oil itself. Whereas, few leafy vegetables can be cooked on low flame with the lid on with no added oil, as they get cooked in the water that gets released from them. If needed, a spoonful of coconut or local oil can be added on top for good taste.

Another mom-daughter conversation

"Just keep the remaining oil in a bottle, we can use it tomorrow morning," said Usha to her daughter.

"We should not reuse it, mom," replied her daughter.

"How can we throw so much oil, it has not even turned black and also the prices have gone up," said Usha with a stern voice?

"You will save money on this, but what about the money you will shell out to lose weight?"

"Is it so bad," asked Usha?

"Yes, it is," replied her daughter as she emptied the oil into the sink.

Oils should never be reused.

Once we have deep-fried certain food items it is best to discard them rather than reuse them. Reason being, the chemical bonds in the oil change after its repeated usage, which makes it unfit for consumption. This is exactly why having samosas and batata vadas (Indian Burger) from roadside vendors may result in fat gain, whereas the occasional home-cooked ones will help you manage your cravings and not cause much harm.

Chapter 15

Do You Have Sweet Tooth?

Diwali hai to mitha jaroori hai (It's festive time so sweets are mandatory.)

Ladki pass hui, mithai lelo (My daughter graduated, it's time to distribute sweets.)

Right from the naming ceremony to the marriage ceremony, there are sweets everywhere. And it's not just special days, our sugar consumption has generally gone up. Look at our meals, right from coffee to ketchup, they all have sugar. This is why there is a spike in people suffering from lifestyle diseases like type 2 diabetes, high blood pressure, heart issues, etc. We know excess sugar is not good for health. Still, what is the reason for its high consumption?

It's addictive, it gives instant gratification, a feeling of pleasure!

Sugar Cycle

- When you get sugar cravings, you extend your hand for a piece of desert.

- As it lands in your hand, your taste buds are activated, and you feel like eating it immediately.

- After taking the first bite, you feel great and you cherish it.

- You get instant gratification, and you keep eating more.

- As it starts digesting, it causes blood sugar levels to go high.

- Insulin plays its part to bring the levels to normal.

- The bigger the portion, the more the insulin used, the higher the fat storage.

- After some time, you feel hungry again and your body craves more sugar (It is addictive.)

The cycle repeats…

As humans, we do things based on our experiences and it applies in the case of sugar consumption too?

E.g.: The last time you were stressed due to your project delays, your colleague told you to have a piece of chocolate and you felt so good after the first bite that you finished the entire bar in no time. Now, it gets stored in your memory that chocolate helps you relieve stress, and the next time you are stressed, you reach out to a chocolate bar.

Sugar offers no nutritional value, hence when you eat biscuits, you've consumed empty calories. *(Calories with no nutrition.)* You are adding calories to your body without getting any nutrition. Plus, you tend to feel hungry in a short time, unlike a roti-sabji meal. (Remember the sugar cycle.)

How sugar negatively impacts your body:

- It is one of the leading causes of many lifestyle-related diseases like diabetes, heart diseases, and obesity.

- It promotes belly fat, so those who say you have only belly fat, check your sugar intake. More the sugar-rich foods you consume, the more the insulin usage, and more the fat storage. (Sugar cycle.)

- It makes you eat more, by impacting leptin resistance. Your brain doesn't get the signals when you are full, leading to overeating.

- It impacts your dental health too.

This list can go on and on. We need to ensure that we consume sugar in limited quantities from the right sources. E.g.: The fruit which you eat has good sugarr, but the sugar found in your desert will harm your body. So, whenever you feel like eating something sweet, have fruit and not a gulab jamun.

Do you get sweet cravings?

Varun, an HR professional had gained a lot of weight in the last few years. He was not a foodie but had got into the habit of eating sweets post-lunch.

Varun: I always feel like having an ice cream post-lunch and that is making me fat.

Can you help?

Me: Are you having a balanced meal?

Varun: I mostly eat roti-sabji.

Me: Do you apply ghee on the roti.

Varun: Should I? Isn't it fattening?

Me: It's not at all fattening and it will help you in dealing with sweet cravings. Also, check the spice level of your food.

Varun: I will do it for my next meal.

Me: And still if you feel like eating sweets, take a pinch of jaggery and fennel post-lunch and you will no longer need ice cream. Also, add coconut to your vegetables and dal and it will help further.

Varun: Sure, I will do this, will keep fennel and jaggery on my desk itself.

A lot of people get these cravings especially after a heavy meal, and then they prefer having an ice cream or some sweet. They blame it on their sweet tooth and some of them also attribute it to their genetics and family. If you want to avoid these cravings, have a balanced meal, and add ghee and coconut to your meals; there are high chances your cravings will reduce.

Where is sugar?

It is not only deserts, chocolates and mithai that contain sugar. Even pizza, burger, pasta, cookies, etc. have a lot of sugar. So, if you consume them regularly, then you should know that your sugar intake is on the higher side. Ketchup, mayos, and most salad dressings too contain a lot of sugar, so do not spoil your healthy salad bowl by adding these sauces. You may be adding just a spoon, but if it's done often, then it's a problem.

Are you someone who says: I prefer multigrain bread, and all the veggies, more olives please (Till here it's perfect.)

But then do you say this too: Add mint mayo and all the sauces!

When you have chaats like bhel, panni puri, etc, there is a lot of sugar added to the chutneys, and the same is the case with doughnuts, ice creams, smoothies, etc. When you say that, *bhaiyaa ek puri free dena, (Give me one puri free)* you should know what you are asking for.

Ek cutting dena, please! (One cup of tea please)

The topic of sugar cannot be completed without talking about tea. Why? We are a tea-drinking nation, where we have bed tea, then breakfast tea, then after reaching office wala tea, then 11:00 a.m. ka tea, then post-lunch ka tea, then 3:00 p.m. ka tea (to stay awake), then office leaving ka tea, then reaching home ka tea, then family ke sath tea and so on.

Here, I am not judging whether the tea is good or bad…that I leave to you, but for every cup *(half cup/ cutting)*, you consume a spoon of sugar. Now imagine if you consume four cups of tea, you are actually taking four spoons of sugar. Now you know why you are not able to reduce your belly, irrespective of doing regular exercises.

Heard about liquid calories?

Beverages have a lot of added sugar; a can of your favourite cola can have up to 7 spoons of sugar. Would you otherwise consume so much sugar? So next time, think twice when you open a can of cola. One last point, I mentioned having fruits to take care of sweet cravings, but avoid having fruit juice, because you lose all the fibre when you juice it.

Quick recap before we hop on to the next chapter:

- Optimise the intake of sugar.

- Have fruits when you get sweet cravings.

- Replace sugar with **jaggery** where required.

- Have ghee, coconut, curd to minimise **sweet cravings.**

- Keep a count on your teacups to avoid sugar intake.

- Stay away from **aerated beverages.**

- Read the **food labels** to understand the amount of sugar.

- Keep handy homemade jaggery and dry fruits based ladoos and have them when you feel like eating dessert.

Chapter 16

Let's Break a Few Fitness Myths

Anchal and her husband Vikrant were discussing a few weight loss stories of their respective colleagues and how they should be serious about their health. Both of them, in their early 30s, were doing good in their corporate carrier but were scoring low on their health.

Anchal: Naomi drinks hot water every day in the office, and she has lost a lot of weight, I will also do the same from tomorrow.

Vikrant: Does it help?

Anchal: Yes, it helps you melt fat!

Vikrant: Wow, that's amazing. I too will start drinking the same.

Anchal: Anyway, we don't have time for exercise, and if hot water helps, then we are sorted.

Ok, I am going to buy two glass bottles as plastic is not good. Do you also want them?

Vikrant: Ya, get for me too and get the customised ones with our names imprinted.

Anchal: Ya, it will look cool too.

And that's how Anchal and her husband started drinking hot water to melt fat. For sure, it helped them consume more water than usual, but the fat melting phenomenon did not happen! There are countless people like Anchal and Vikrant who tend to believe in a few such myths, let's take time to debunk them.

What is a myth?

It is a false belief, which we follow, thinking it is true. In the above example, it was about hot water melting fat.

Similarly, there are more, let's look at them one by one.

Myth: Six-pack equals fitness

When I talk to youngsters, one common thing I hear: I need six-pack abs. For them, that is equivalent to fitness and they are ready to put in whatever effort is required. It has become a fashion statement nowadays and is flaunted more than your bank balance. But donning a six-pack does not guarantee that you are fit! Everyone has it. *(You can check now.)* Just that it is covered by a layer (s) of fat. Once you shed the overall body fat, it will be visible. Talking about fat, like we said earlier, there is an ideal range for it, and if you fit in that range, it is a good sign of your fitness, along with your non-scale parameters.

It's around 15 % for males and 25% for females and it varies according to age but consider these numbers as ballpark figures for good health.

For you to have those 6 pack abs, you need to further reduce your fat % to less than 10% or even more. It is not that easy and healthy to reduce fat to this extent. (*Remember our body needs it.*)

How come these actors and bodybuilders flaunt it?

- The first thing is the need to have it for their profession.

- Second, they have been exercising regularly for long, and not just for three to four months.

- Third and most important, they flaunt these packs for a particular period when they are working for a particular movie or are on stage for a performance and not year-round. (*Although a few are an exception to this, here we are talking about 80% of the population where you and I belong.*)

Hence it works well for them.

Is it not possible?

It is and for that, you need to work on your fitness the right way and follow all that we have covered till now consistently.

Myth: You can choose the areas where you want to lose fat.

Let me tell you about Kaushal, a chef by profession working in a 5-star hotel in Delhi. We were talking about how to get a flat stomach.

Kaushal: I am fit, just this paunch you know. I have started doing 100 crunches daily, am sure this will go.

Me: A 100 crunches daily! Are you kidding me!

Kaushal: Ya, I plan to take it to 200 over a week and then 300 and even 400.

Abhi to flat stomach karke hi rahega, he further said. (Now I will ensure that I get a flat stomach.)

Me: Sirf crunches karke nahi banta flat stomach (You can't get six packs just by doing crunches) Kaushal, you need to work on your bigger muscle groups: Legs, back, chest and take care of your meals.

Kaushal: That's all perfect, koi fat nahi hai, (there is no fat) it is just this stomach.

Abhi jaha pe fat hai, wohi pe jada exercise hona chaiyee na, he questioned? (Shouldn't we exercise those body parts where there is more fat?)

Me: Look, it doesn't work that way. You cannot pick and choose the body parts where you want to reduce fat, you need to look at reducing overall body fat.

Kaushal: What are you saying? I am doing it for the past three weeks.

Me: Did you drop any inches from your waistline?

Kaushal: No, but it will reduce in a couple of weeks more.

Me: It won't, tell me one more thing, do you get lower back pain?

Kaushal: Yes, when I do above 30 counts, I start getting back pain.

Me: So still, you continue?

Kaushal: Of course, No pain – no gain. Thoda to sahan karna padega, body bananeka hai to (I am fine to take some suffering to get fit).

I smiled and said, let me explain.

Our body tends to store fat in different areas, and it can differ from person to person. Some store it in arms, some in the upper back, some in thighs, some over hips, and so on. Hence the focus should be on reducing overall body fat by doing compound exercises and eating right and not targeting the stubborn body part. When you do something like 100 crunches, you are just putting extreme pressure on your abdomen and back muscles and there are high chances you will sprain it. In the end, your muscles get overworked and they give up; the fat does not budge.

Myth: Walking is the best exercise for fat loss

Walking makes us feel fresh, particularly if it is done early morning in an open space. Breathing fresh air lifts our mood and makes us happy. It also enhances blood circulation throughout the body. As opposed to sitting and being sedentary, it is always better to walk and be active.

But if your goal is fat loss, then it may not be sufficient. If you recollect, we mentioned a relationship between OHR and fat loss. When you walk, your heart rate doesn't rise much and hence doesn't help in losing fat unlike other forms of strength training exercises. You see so many people walking in the garden for an hour daily, but still, they have a paunch.

So, should you not walk?

You should, but do not just do that, get involved in other exercises too. Walking is suitable for those who cannot do any other exercises due to injury or some health condition. It is better that they walk than not do anything at all. And for those looking at fat loss, don't waste time walking. (*We are so busy.*) Use that time to do strength training, support it with the right meals and you will see results.

Myth: Warm water melts fat.

We mentioned Anchal's story that she started drinking hot water to lose fat and it did not help her. Let's talk about this myth.

I know so many working professionals carrying thermos to the office to fill it with hot water and drink it throughout the day. I have seen people literally standing in a queue near the water dispenser to fill hot water, first thing in the morning. Not all of them fill it with the intent to lose fat, but most do. While warm water (*not hot*) is generally good for your health and throat, it will not help you lose fat. So, stay away from unnecessarily gulping hot water. Drink it as per your requirement.

Myth: The more you sweat, the more weight you lose.

I tend to sweat even while standing, so does it mean I am losing weight?

Unfortunately, No!

Sweating is the body's mechanism to adjust body temperature.

While doing cardio exercises you sweat a lot (*recollect aerobic exercises*) and you burn calories too, while doing strength training, you may not sweat much, but you still use your muscle and lose fat. (R*ecollect after-burn.*)

Again, in strength training, there are exercises like jumping squats, walking lunges which will make you sweat a lot, while some core sequences like planks and scissors, do not make you sweat much, but it still works very well on your muscles. Hence, sweating is not an indication of weight loss.

Sit in a room in Mumbai for 15 minutes without a fan in the month of May, and you will sweat like crazy, but then understand your body is not losing fat. A few people purposely close the windows or switch off the Acs or fans during a workout just to sweat! Their logic is, if and only if they sweat, they feel like they have done a workout. It is actually counterproductive and hinders an effective workout by tiring you out during the session.

Myth: More time in the gym = better body.

Rahil wanted to lose weight to go on a vacation and that's how he got in touch with me. He used to work out a few years back, but the last few years he got tied up with academics.

Rahil: What is the duration of your exercise session?

Me: Around 45 minutes…

Rahil: Just 45 minutes! I used to work out for 1–1.5 hours in the gym, can I get a longer session?.

Me: Sure Rahil, why don't you come for a trial this Saturday, we are doing a full body workout.

Rahil: Looks good, I will be there.

On Saturday, our session started at 8:00 a.m. and Rahil joined at the right time. We had just finished two to three sequences and he interrupted.

Rahil: I can't go any further, I am tired.

Me: Please take a break and join us back towards the end, for the cool-down session.

Post-session, he gave me a call and said it was a real workout. He could not do much.

Me: Rahil, on day 1 it is expected that you do only 15 minutes of the low-intensity workout and gradually you build stamina to do the entire session.

Rahil: Sure.

Quality vs Quantity again!

More than the duration of exercise, how you do it is more important. You will often see people spending two hours in the gym, but most of the time they are either talking to someone or doing a J walk on a treadmill for 45–60 minutes.

Recall what we discussed about OHR, HIIT, and how it helps you.

Also, your body needs the energy to exercise and it starts draining out gradually. And if you have not consumed the right pre-workout meal, you will lose energy in the initial 10–15 minutes, forget 60 minutes. There is absolutely no point in pushing yourself when you are drained out. You may end up pushing the wrong muscle leading to an injury. So, exercising for 30–45 minutes with the right intensity will help. Anything beyond 60 is not worth it (unless you are a pro).

Myth: Not eating post-workout helps in fat loss

We discussed in one of the previous chapters how protein plays an important role in post-workout muscle recovery. Also, as you exercise, your glycogen levels are depleted and need replenishment. A fruit followed by the right protein-rich meal takes care of both. If you do not eat post-workout, thinking that the body will burn fat, it's not going to work in your favour. Your body will crave energy, and it will result in muscle loss.

Fat is **FILO (First In Last out)** and doesn't go by mere fasting. What goes is your hard-earned muscle. Hence never fast or starve yourself after your workout.

Myth: Exercise can compensate for a bad diet

Another conversation between gym buddies Omkar and Kian.

Omkar: Let's have wada pav (Indian Burger).

Kian: But that has a lot of calories, and we just had a workout, let's eat something healthy.

Omkar: Doesn't matter, we did almost 90 minutes of workout and have burnt a lot of calories. Besides, we will do it again tomorrow, so a wada pav will not harm us.

Kian: Alright, let's have it. (And they both binged on wada pav. No one can eat just one ☺.)

Exercise can never compensate for a bad diet. Let's understand by taking the same example:

- One exercise session will help you burn around 150 – 200 calories, depending on your intensity.

- One wada pav will add 400–450 calories to your body.

Now it's not rocket science to understand that any excess calories not used by the body will result in fat gain. And it's not just about calories, look at how you are getting your calories.

If maximum calories are coming from fat, then this food needs to be consumed sparingly.

Another thing is exercise contributes around 30% to your fitness and your meals play an even bigger role. Hence, if you just focus on the former, you will not get the desired results.

Myth: Detox drinks are mandatory for fat loss

Detox drinks will help you improve your digestion, or soothe your throat, but it doesn't influence fat loss. Our body is not like the carburettor of your bike where you put good oil *(detox water)* from above, open the outlet and all the waste is drained out. In fact, we have a natural detox system, we have to just eat right, consume a good amount of fibre, drink enough water and the body will take care on its own.

You can still consume these drinks, but don't link them to fat loss and don't make sour faces while consuming them. *(I know someone who drinks Karela juice every day, but still carries a paunch.)*

Instead, once in two weeks, have a fruit and salad day, where you eat only fresh fruits and vegetables, and you will feel light.

Myth: I play with my kid, that's more than enough exercise for me.

Playing with your kid is always fun, but don't confuse it with exercise, unless you are playing a sport. Think about the exercise principles of OHR, aerobic, and anaerobic energy system, progressive overload, HIIT. If none of them is followed, then it is not equivalent to exercise. Nowadays, many parents cannot play due to some pain or fatigue and regular exercise will make you stronger to play a sport with your kid. I know someone who started exercising when she realised, she couldn't play with her five-year-old kid.

Myth: I do household work, so I do not need to exercise

It is still better than being sedentary, but to qualify it as exercise, think along the same lines *(exercise principles)*. Some activities like shifting heavy objects do involve muscle movements, but not all. Exercising regularly will help you in doing household activities efficiently.

Myth: Counting calories is a good practice

If you eat more calories than your body needs, you gain weight and if you eat fewer calories than what you need, you lose weight. It is not that simple. It's equally important to know about the source of calories.

E.g.: There is no point in eating calories from cookies, even if the calorie count may fit your requirement. Whereas, if it comes from good carbs, lean protein, or good fats, it serves the purpose. Also, counting calories looks feasible for the initial few weeks, but doing it regularly is not feasible.

I am sure this information will help you in your fitness journey. Next time, when you hear any of these myths, please educate them with the right knowledge. Stay tuned, as we talk about lifestyle in the next chapter.

Chapter 17
Fitness Lifestyle

Let me tell you about Kirti. She is a single mother, and she works as an Operations Manager with an FMCG organisation. A hectic job and a growing daughter kept her so tied up, that she couldn't look after her own health. She had piled up a lot of weight which caused her several health issues. She was desperate to lose weight.

Kirti: Can you give me a plan by which I can get fit in 30 days? I will follow everything you say, right from exercise to a strict diet.

Me: In one month, I can help you adapt to a healthy lifestyle.

Kirti: I already have a good job, a premium sedan, own a house, go on vacations, and shop for anything I want… so what else do I need?

Me: I am not talking about your social status, but the way you spend your day in terms of your eating habits, your meal timings, your activities, your social outings which influence your health.

Kirti: But I just want to lose weight, can you not give me a magical diet plan.

Me: There is no such plan Kirti and if it exists, then I am not aware of it.

Kirti: I have a couple of friends who lost weight last year by following one such diet.

Me: Call it a crash diet. Tell me one thing Kirti, if you have seen their results, then why don't you follow the same diet, it will give you the same results too?

Kirti: That was the initial plan, but when I met one of them last week, he had again gained weight.

Me: That is what I mean Kirti, there is no such diet plan which will give you quick results. And even if you manage it initially, will you able to sustain it for a lifetime?

Kirti: No.

Me: Your fitness is not just a temporary weight loss to be achieved in a month, it is a lifelong activity. So, the steps you take should be such that you'd be able to do it for life.

Kirti: That's the lifestyle you mean.

Me: Exactly, now let us work on analysing your lifestyle and making changes as required.

Kirti: How?

Me: I'll give you a few tips, which will help you do that, have a look.

Tip: Say no to Crash Diets:

Crash diets/fad diets are available everywhere. We saw how Kirti's friend lost weight due to crash dieting and gained it back too quickly. A crash diet is a very low-calorie diet intended for quick weight loss. Results of this type of diet are short-lived and you tend to gain the lost weight once you stop it.

Let's take an example of one such diet:

Breakfast – Cornflakes

Lunch – One chapati and vegetables

Snacks – One glass of apple juice

Dinner – Soup/salad (Don't look for more, that's it.)

Some of you will just faint looking at it, isn't it too low?

Some people may be eating all of it in one meal!

Ask yourself, will it give you the required energy for your daily activities, forget workouts. And if you exercise on such a diet, it can be catastrophic. We have seen how pre- and post-workout meals are essential for effective workouts and recovery. In the absence of it, you are just losing muscle.

Such meals may give you short-term results, but you cannot follow such plans for a long time. Also, the initial weight you lose is more of muscle and water loss; your fat stores are not touched. By now, we know that losing fat and adding lean muscle is our goal and not the other way round.

Results of such diets are:

Weight loss (temporary) + No fat loss + Muscle loss + No strength + Bad posture + Probably bad digestion too.

Hence the first rule of a healthy lifestyle is to *say no to crash diets.*

Tip: It's more than just 40 minutes of workout

Your workout is less than an hour of your day and it plays a role in making you stronger.

But if you think that since your workout is done, you can be sedentary for the remaining 23 hours *(minus the sleep time)*, then it will not help.

You need to remain active throughout the day and by that, I don't mean you should be working out twice a day. You should be moving and not be sitting in one place. If your work demands to be seated at a desk, ensure that you take breaks every hour.

Why these breaks are needed and how they help:

- Sitting at a desk increases the pressure on your spine, causing pain. When you take a break and walk or stretch, it reduces the risks of such sprains and pain.

- Sitting for long hours impacts blood circulation, causing numbness in the legs. When you get up and walk, it ensures blood circulation.

- Working on a computer for long not only puts pressure on your back but also your wrist, hence taking a break and doing palm stretches or wrist rotations help. Wrist injuries take time to heal, so protect your wrist.

- When you sit for long, or when you plan to sit for long, there are chances you may keep snacks like chips and beverages handy at your desk. While working, we do not realise how much we eat, and this can compromise your fitness routine.

- Stretching or doing mobility drills will help you keep your muscles and joints active. Take a break for a minimum of five minutes every hour you sit and do a few stretches.

Refer to our Facebook post for chair-based exercises, which can be done in five minutes. *(Link in the appendix section.)*

Tip: Bring Variety

Eating five to six portion-controlled meals will help you meet the nutrition requirement. But if you are going to eat the same food every day, then you may get bored. Bring variety in your meals and it will help you stay aligned.

Depending on the time availabe, make some interesting curd-based salads *(they are easy to make)*.

There is a huge variety of green leafy vegetables, pulses, legumes which are healthy, add them to your meals than just eating spinach, potatoes, and paneer.

Do try different cooking methods like grill, sauté, tandoor, boiled to bring a different taste to everyday food. Foods like panner or mushroom can be cooked on the grill or just sautéed in five to 10 minutes. Boiled chana with a mix of onion, tomatoes, chillies is a wholesome meal.

Add good quality spices in required quantities to give flavour to food. Black pepper, chat masalas can be added to salads and fruit plates to enhance their taste.

Look for healthy, interesting recipes and try them out on weekends.

E.g.: Take a pan, put one spoon ghee, add 2–3 pieces of panner, sprinkle salt/pepper, and cook for five minutes. It is quick and tasty.

Additionally, take a chapati/roti, add the panner pieces, add chutney if handy, make a roll.

It will taste good and provide you with the right nutrition quickly.

And the last one, do indulge in cheat meals occasionally.

Tip: Look at Your Posture

You can increase your height, if you focus on your posture, try doing it as you read this.

Not just that, bad posture is also related to neck and back pain, hence maintaining the right posture is beneficial. When you feel some tightness in your back, try sitting in a proper posture, you may get some relief.

Exercise and posture are interdependent:

Exercise helps you improve your posture by making your muscles stronger, whereas exercising in the wrong posture can lead to injuries. Swinging your back or extensive movements of the neck are two of the most common exercise mistakes. Doing core workouts help in improving the posture, hence include them as part of your plan. A weak core puts pressure on the spine leading to bad posture.

While we focus on meals and exercises, posture is most often ignored. No wonder you see people with bulging biceps and broad shoulders with rounded backs. The problem is, when you get into a poor posture every day, your body structure slowly changes and adapts to it, resulting in pain.

The good part is you can improve your posture:

- Exercise regularly and focus on the right form.

- Stand in front of a mirror and practice the right posture by keeping the spine erect and not slouching. Do this for three to five minutes daily and your posture will improve.

- To check your mobile, bring it in front of your face rather than looking down.

- While sitting at a work desk, ensure that your feet are flat on the surface, your back is not slouched, and the computer screen is in line with your eyesight. *(Use laptop stands as required.)*

- Take a break every hour and stretch your body.

Practice these things for consecutive 21 days, and you will get into good posture.

Tip: Try Different Exercises

The way you should try different food options, you should bring a variety of exercises too. Doing the same exercise variations can cause boredom and beats the purpose of progressive overload. You need to challenge and surprise your body by trying different exercises.

- If you are into functional training, go for a swim once a week or a run.

- If you are a gym-goer, play a sport on a Sunday.

- If you are into strength training, then do yoga once a week.

- Try kickboxing, martial arts, krav maga, boxing, or cycling. You may take time to learn, but your body will slowly adapt. Krav maga and functional training go hand in hand. The punches, kicks and grabs you learn in the former can be added to the HIIT sequence in the latter.

E.g. – Build a circuit of 20 straight punches + 10 jumping jacks; 20 uppercuts + 10 mummy kicks; 20 roundhouses + 10 sprints. Repeat till fatigue. This is an amazing HIIT sequence.

Do ensure that you follow the exercise rules we discussed earlier (Warm-up, cool-down, meals.)

Tip: Mental Fitness

Stress, if not managed well, can play a spoiler. Starting your day with 10 minutes of deep breathing followed by five minutes of meditation will help you manage it. I have been doing this for two years now, and my mornings are blissful.

Try this:

- Wake up at 5:30 a.m. (*You need to sleep at least by 10:30 p.m.*)

- Post your morning routine, drink warm water. (*I prefer adding a few spices, aloe, honey to hot water.*)

- Take a yoga mat and head to an open area. (*I prefer going to the terrace.*)

- Locate a space, sit cross-legged or the way you are comfortable.

- Look at the sky as you take a sip of water.

- Do deep breathing for 10 minutes:

  - Take a deep breath on the count of 1 to 7.

  - Hold your breath for 4 counts and release.

  - Take a break for 4 counts and then breathe again.

- Post this, do a five-minute meditation session.

- If you have more time, plan your day too.

The above practice can be done in as little as 15 to 20 minutes and it gives a lot of positive energy. And when the start itself is so good, the day will be amazing.

I never miss this morning ritual wherever I am, and it just makes my day.

Tip: Visualisation

Add another five minutes to the above routine and do this:

- Sit in a comfortable position and keep your eyes closed.

- Visualise that you have achieved the desired fitness levels (*as per your fitness goal*).

- With the same mindset, imagine that you go in to work wearing nice, fit clothes, eat healthy meals, exercise with amazing intensity, finish your dinner early, and sleep on time. You can even think about the exercise routines you do, your exercise wear, what exactly you will eat for lunch, and how tall you stand maintaining the right posture. The deeper you go; the closer you will feel towards your goal.

- This works very well when done consecutively for 90 days.

Tip: Muscle Meditation

If mornings are blissful, you will have a wonderful day. Once your day is done, it's time to get to bed. But some people experience fatigue, tiredness and are not able to sleep properly. If you are sleep deprived, then your exercise and meals do not help.

Doing muscle mediation helps you get rid of work and other stress and allows you to sleep peacefully. This can be done in as little as 20 minutes, but if you can spend more time (30 to 45 minutes) it will help. This must be done once you are ready to sleep. So, make your bed, get into your sleepwear, keep water handy, dim the lights, and start with the session. It is so peaceful that five out of 10 people sleep in the first 15 minutes. Try doing it for a week and let me know your feedback.

In the appendix, I have provided my YouTube link for a muscle meditation session.

Tip: Lymphatic System

Do you often feel unwell, or do you experience a feeling of heaviness? Then, you need to know about the lymphatic system which plays a major role in building our immunity. The lymphatic system is 80% of our health and a huge piece of beauty and it determines whether we wake up fresh and beautiful, or sleepy and tired. No, I am not trying to complicate things, but you all need to know about it.

Lymph is the fluid that flows throughout the lymphatic system; it must flow freely to ensure that waste products do not build up in the tissues. When this is disturbed, up to 80% of the harmful substances are not filtered out but get accumulated in the intercellular space where they gradually sprout with fibres of connective tissue (fibrosis) and clog up all the channels.

Poor waste removal in the lymphatic system can affect almost any part of your body. When your lymph vessels become congested, you may experience:

- Fatigue

- Bloating

- Water retention

- Stiffness, especially in the morning

- Itchy and dry skin

- Cellulite

- Stubborn weight gain

- Chronic sinusitis, sore throats, colds, and ear issues

- Cold hands and feet and much more

Lack of exercise, intake of junk food, and a sedentary lifestyle affects this system badly. There are various methods like dry brushing, hot and cold showers, etc to enhance the lymphatic system, **but the best way is to change your lifestyle**.

Tip: Plan for Required Resources

If you fail to plan, you plan to fail, said the great Benjamin Franklin.

This holds equally true in your fitness journey, hence plan your life well.

You will need a few resources, so keep the list handy:

- Vegetable and Fruit vendors.

- Healthy meal recipes if you plan to cook.

- Meal providers if you plan to buy meals.

- Meal plans.

- Gyms/Fitness centres.

- Personal trainers if you plan to have one.

- Equipment/tools if you plan to workout at home.

- Fitness accessories: shoes, tracks, tees, grips, bands, etc.

- Massage centres.

- Doctors/physio in case of injuries.

You may also want to decide on responsibilities:

- Who will cook meals? – If you are dependent on your family, tell them in advance when and what type of meals you need as they may have their priorities. If you have a cook, clearly instruct him about your preferences and meal timings. If you have any specific recipes, do share them with your cook.

- Who will buy the groceries? – If you are staying with your family and you expect them to buy it, then communicate it to them accordingly. Assuming that someone will get it, will not help.

- Who will give you reminders? – If you need a meal or wake up reminders, either tell someone or invest in a tool.

- And also, who will take the stick? – If you go off track or are not following the plan, then there should be someone to question you *(It may sound strict, but at times it helps.)*

A healthy lifestyle is what will make you fit for life and practising these tips will help you in the long run.

Chapter 18
No More Broken Hearts

Nikita was talking to her colleague Cruz over breakfast. She was in shock over the demise of her friend.

Nikita: But he was just 28, is this the age to get a heart attack?

Cruz: It's no longer the case that only once you cross a certain age there are chances of a heart attack. I know a friend whose brother was just 26. And that too, he was into exercises and sports.

Nikita: This is shocking, then what is the point of exercising?

Cruz: Just exercising will not help, it's also about how we manage other things too.

Nikita: That's right.

The number of heart attacks has gone up in the past few years and it is no longer relevant only to a particular age group. Even young people suffer from heart conditions and a bad lifestyle is a major contributor. We focus on building the visible muscles like biceps, shoulders chest, and forget about the most important muscular organ, our heart. But the good part is, we do not need any separate exercises for the heart, and our very own strength training and cardio exercises work well.

When you do strength training, it not just strengthens your chest, back, and other muscles, but also your heart, by making its walls stronger and helping it function effectively. This, along with cardio exercises, work very well in improving heart health. Refer to the chapter on exercise to know more about the different forms of exercise.

Other than exercise, eating habits also influence heart health. Regular consumption of high fat, sugary foods and alcohol clogs the arteries impacting blood circulation and the functioning of the heart. Eating a balanced meal with added good fats works in favour of the heart.

Temporary taste on your tongue can lead to permanent side effects on your heart. Hence, beware of what you eat. Cheat meals consumed occasionally are not a problem though.

Stress is another factor that impacts your heart. Exercises, deep breathing and mediation help you beat stress. High levels of cortisol from long-term stress can increase blood cholesterol, triglycerides, blood sugar, and blood pressure leading to heart diseases. Even if you get stressed over trivial things, it can impact blood flow to the heart. Stress and smoking are related, and the effects of smoking are known enough. (Refer to the chapter on stress for details)

Quick tips:

- Consume less sugar, salt, bad fats and have more **balanced meals.**

- Be aware of **packaged food** *(Read nutrition labels.)*

- Never miss your **breakfast.**

- Do **exercise regularly.**

- **Stay active**, take stairs as feasible.

- Say no to **smoking.**

- Minimise intake of **alcohol.**

- Manage your **stress.**

- **Assess** your health regularly.

- Take a **break** *(Go for vacations.)*

- **Spend time** with friends and family.

And the last one, take things easy, do not hassle too much over too many things.

Chapter 19

For The Records

Ramya is a college student and is very social. She ensures that she participates in all the events and that has made her gain a lot of weight. She does exercise but keeps taking breaks often.

Ramya: I have been exercising regularly, but still, my weight has not moved much.

Me: Are you regular?

Ramya: Yes.

Me: But I saw your vacation pictures on IG.

Ramya: Ya, that was only two weeks, but before that, I was regular.

Me: If I am not wrong, I also met you at Piyush's wedding in Surat.

Ramya: Ya, that was only for three days.

Me: But both these events were this month itself!

Ramya: Right, but the remaining days, I did my workouts

Me: Are you 100% sure?

Ramya: I think yes...let me recollect... I may have missed a couple of sessions.

Me: Do you maintain an exercise journal?

Ramya: What's that?

Me: Do you check your credit card statement regularly?

Ramya: Yes, every time I pay my bill. I first check the statement.

Me: Does it help?

Ramya: Yes, it does help me know where I have made unnecessary spends.

Me: Good, let's extend the same to your fitness.

Let me explain:

We live a busy life managing multiple things, right from work, family, finances, travel, and health. Sometimes, one thing takes priority over the other and we end up not doing things as planned. So, making a note of important things helps.

If you look at Ramya's case, she was worried about her results and she also assumed that she was regular in her workouts but was not sure about it. Had she maintained an exercise journal, she would have been sure about it.

It's not a big task to maintain it, but it needs practice:

Exercise Journal:

Sr No	Date	Day	Exercise	Remarks
1	06-06-12	Monday	Chest – Triceps	Any specific remarks about Sets/ Reps
2	08-06-12	Wednesday	Legs	

Your fitness is also influenced by what you eat, so tracking meal details will also help.

Am I asking for too much?

Trust me it works ☺.

This can be captured in a simple format:

6 – June, Monday:

7:00 a.m. – Dry fruits

7:45 a.m. – Poha + one boiled egg

10:15 a.m. – Apple

12:45 p.m. – two chapatis + Brinjal curry + Buttermilk

3:30 p.m. – Green tea

4:45 p.m. – Makahana

6:30 pm – One chapati + Methi vegetable

8:45 p.m. – Warm milk.

Or you can use the exercise journal and capture both things simultaneously. Ensure that you capture the right data each time you make an entry.

Exercise and Meal Journal

Sr No	Date	Day	Exercise	Meals	Remarks
1	06-06-12	Monday	Chest – Triceps	7:00 am – Dry fruits 7.45 am – Poha + 1 boiled egg 10.15 am – Apple 12.45 pm – 2 chapati + Brinjal curry + Buttermilk 3.30 pm – Green tea 4:45 pm – Makahana 6:30 pm – 1 chapati + Methi vegetable 8.45pm – Warm milk	Any specific remarks about Sets/Reps
2	08-06-12	Wednesday	Legs	<add details>	

It will take not more than 30 seconds to update this daily.

Don't just capture this data, use it the right way:

At the end of the week or month, do look at it and check how many sessions you did, how many times you missed your meals, and how many cheat meals were included.

This can help you compare your progress in line with your goals.

This journal can be maintained in a book or a spreadsheet for easy access.

Chapter 20
Do You Switch Off?

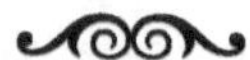

Vishwa, an MBA student likes to stay fit and he does keep a tab on his meals. We were discussing the role of sleep in fitness. I made him stand on a scale to check his body composition parameters.

Vishwa: Your machine is not working properly. I exercise regularly, and my meals are home-cooked, still, this machine says my visceral fat is 17%. I just cannot believe it.

Me: What time do you sleep?

Vishwa: It is not fixed, depends on my assignments, but you know I just need five hours of sleep, unlike others who sleep for eight to nine hours. I feel it's a waste of time.

Me: And why do you feel so?

Vishwa: We just have 24 hours a day and if I sleep for eight to nine hours, then how will I get time to do other things?

Me: Why do you feel that five hours of sleep is sufficient for you?

Vishwa: I cannot sleep more than that, and I have to rush to the gym too.

Me: That is the reason for your high visceral fat.

Vishwa: What has sleep to do with this fat? I burn a lot of calories in the gym every day.

Me: Even then, your number is on the higher side, so don't you think something is not right?

Vishwa: I know if you do not get enough sleep, you may feel tired. But does it also impact visceral fat%?

Me: It does. What time do you sleep?

Vishwa: I get to bed by midnight and sleep by 2:00 a.m.

Me: I did not get you, what do you do for two hours.

Vishwa: That is my *me time*. Throughout the day, I do not get time to look at my social media feeds and to watch my favourite Netflix series. So, I spend some time on it.

Me: It's not your me time, but your sleep time Vishwa. This is why your visceral fat is high. Sleep on time, get a good seven to eight hours of sleep and you will drop this fat%.

Vishwa: Will it work for sure?

Me: Try it and get back to me in a month, my machine will tell you then.

Not sure, whether he liked it, but he gave me a call 1.5 months later.

Vishwa: "Sleeping on time has done wonders for me. My exercise performance has gone up and I feel more energetic. I am sure my visceral fat% would have also gone down."

Me: Congratulations, how did you manage this.

Vishwa: I just did one thing, I switch off my cell by 11:00 p.m., and this has helped.

Me: Do tell your friends too and help them get fit.

Vishwa: Sure

Sleep is the most important and often overlooked aspect of fitness. Good sleep can do wonders for your body, right from feeling fresh to helping you lose weight. It's a natural healer.

Whereas bad sleep can affect your overall health and increase the chances of heart ailments, blood pressure, diabetes, and obesity.

Sleep and Fat Loss go Hand in Hand

There can be multiple reasons for this correlation, but I want to keep it simple:

If you sleep less, you have less energy to exercise and to make the right food choices, this impacts fat loss. Additionally, the more time you are awake, you tend to eat more. Recall the late-night fridge visits to munch on chocolates and gulab jamuns.

And for the ones, who need details:

If you do not get the required sleep, cortisol levels (stress hormones) are not controlled effectively which causes high blood sugar, leading to obesity.

Do you recollect a discussion on leptin?

It is an appetite-regulating hormone that tells your brain that your stomach is full, so you stop eating. Lack of sleep does not allow leptin to function effectively, which may lead to overeating. Imagine you keep on eating bigger portions! Hence, sleeping for seven to eight hours, preferably between 10:00 p.m. – 6:00 a.m. is beneficial.

But I sleep longer over the weekends to finish my quota, said Piyusha.

This is not like a camel hump, where you can store sleep hours and use it as required. This is about your daily sleep which plays an important role. You just cannot sleep on the weekends to make up for your lack of sleep during the week, I replied.

Weekend sleeping has become a common practice, mostly among working professionals. Late-night calls, travel time, and family commitments don't allow people to sleep well during weekdays. Hence many try to catch up on their sleep during the weekends. But it's not a good practice as the body needs rest on a daily basis.

So, is sleeping more on weekends bad? No, if you want to rest more and feel relaxed, but do not use it to compensate for your weekday sleep.

How to Sleep Better?

Tip: It's always better to sleep at a fixed time:

Observe your sleep schedule for a week, then fix a schedule and stick to it. This makes your body get used to a particular schedule and allows it to relax and slow down as you come closer to the sleep time. Our system is smart, it adapts to a routine gradually, but if you keep changing routines, our system doesn't appreciate it much. This is one of the reasons for not getting sound sleep. You must have heard about jet lag!

Tip: Finish your dinner before 7:00 p.m., so you can be in bed by 10:00 p.m.

Just like you cannot exercise effectively after a heavy meal, similarly, undigested food in the stomach doesn't allow you to sleep. When you sleep you need more blood circulation in your brain, which is impacted due to undigested food. Hence, keeping a gap of a minimum of three hours post-dinner helps.

We have been talking about finishing dinners before 7:00 p.m. and if you do that, you can doze off by 10:00 p.m.

Tip: Avoid gadgets at least 60 minutes before you sleep

We've had the concept of night lamps or yellow lights or dim lights for ages. Reason being, the lower the white or blue light, the better the chances of getting sleep. Mobiles, laptops, and other gadgets emit a lot of bright light, which doesn't allow your body to relax. Hence, make it a practice to keep gadgets away at least an hour before bedtime.

You can always read a book or listen to soothing music to induce sleep.

Tip: Create a soothing environment, use curtains, and eye masks as needed

You need to make your room look nice to sleep better. I know a few blessed souls who can sleep anywhere, but I am talking about people like you and me. If there is a lot of light coming from the street or if there are people around it can impact your sleep. Using dark curtains and eye masks will help you sleep.

Tip: Make your bed, first thing in the morning.

A good practice is to make your bed as soon as you wake up. You may wonder how this helps? Imagine you come home stressed and tired and want to sleep. And you see your bed ready, how good you will feel.

Now imagine, after coming home, you realise that you have to make your bed. Wouldn't it put off your mood? The tasks which take just five minutes in the morning will look like a herculean task now!

So, it's a good practice to keep your bed ready, so you can get into slumber quickly. It also helps you start your day in a disciplined manner. (*Cleaning your mess is the best thing you can do.*)

Tip: Avoid loud sounds and keep the room at a comfortable temperature.

We are aware of the impact of sound pollution on our health. Exposure to loud sounds during sleep can be a distractor. One, it prevents you from falling asleep initially and two, it creates restlessness in sleep. Insulate your doors and windows using curtains and other soundproofing mechanisms. Switch off electronics like TV, mobiles, or put them in silent mode.

If you plan to sleep in crowded places when you travel, wear earplugs. *(Make sure they are soft and flexible.)* Still, if there is a disturbing sound, playing light *(meditative type)* music helps.

If someone disturbs your early morning sleep, it can be irritating, hence tell your milk and newspaper delivery persons not to ring the doorbell.

Room temperature too impacts your sleep, hence maintain a soothing and comfortable temperature in your room, not too hot and not too cold either. It will still differ from person to person, as some prefer to keep it cold while others just can't sleep at that temperature.

Tip: Practice muscle meditation.

There is enough evidence to support that mediation helps induce sleep. I have been practising muscle meditation for two years now, and it has given me good benefits. I have covered that in one of the previous chapters and will also include a link to one of my sessions.

Tip: Exercise regularly.

"If you get tired, you will sleep early, hence go out and play." This is what mothers tell their kids, mostly during summer vacations. That holds true even for adults. Don't be sedentary, exercise for good sleep. It also improves your mood and stabilises your mind, making you sleep better. Don't exercise too close to sleep time, as it might interfere.

Tip: Try a warm bath before bed.

There was a time when our ancestors used to do it, but I'm not sure it is practised today. Hot water helps in changing your body's core temperature so that you go to bed with a lower temperature. It is also associated with relaxation, which will help you sleep peacefully.

Tip: Avoid drinking a lot of water before sleep to avoid making washroom visits.

Imagine you are in deep sleep and someone wakes you, how do you feel? Similarly, washroom visits at night can be irritating.

I know a friend who had to do an MRI scan to diagnose the headache he had been going through for almost three months. Multiple visits to a doctor and numerous reports pointed out that everything was well inside. The only reason for his headache (he realised later) was a break in his sleep due to regular washroom visits at night. He had got into the habit of drinking warm water at night (I hope it was not for fat loss) which urged him to pee in the middle of the night. This happened for almost a month and one day he got this throbbing headache in the office and it stayed for almost three months. He started sleeping right and his headache just vanished in two weeks.

And once there is a break, getting back to sleep can also be a task for a few. Hence consuming minimal water close to sleep time will help.

Tip: Avoid consumption of caffeine late in the day.

Caffeine is a stimulant and makes us feel fresh. Why would you want to feel fresh and alert when you want to get to bed? Hence avoid its consumption post 6:00 p.m., though I know a few who can sleep right after consuming a cup of coffee.

Tip: Avoid or reduce daytime naps, though I believe a power nap of 15 minutes helps.

If you are someone who finds it difficult to sleep at night, then first start being active and second avoid any naps throughout the day. We will talk about power naps later in the chapter.

Tip: Avoid any work-related discussions close to sleep time, this keeps the mind occupied with thoughts and ideas and interferes with sleep.

"I am telling you six nights will not be sufficient, we need at least eight nights for this vacation," said Golu to his wife, while in the bed.

"You are still awake!" asked his wife. "It's been more than 45 minutes since you went to bed."

"I tried sleeping, but this thought doesn't go off my mind," he replied.

How many of you have gone through this situation? I am sure there are many! Hence avoid any discussions which will creep through your mind while you sleep. Now I know when people say, "Jyada paisa nahi chaiyee, sirf raat ko neend aani chaiyee." What they mean is, what is the point of earning so much money if your mind is occupied with thoughts and doesn't allow you to sleep.

Stages of Sleep

- Non-REM (Non-Rapid Eye Movement)

- REM (Rapid Eye Movement)

There is enough written about these stages, to keep it short:

It's a transition from feeling drowsy – light sleep – deep sleep.

As we go through these stages, our heart rate, breathing pattern, eye movements, body temperature, brain activity slows down and allows us to sleep peacefully.

Do you feel irritated or hyper or you get mood swings?

Check if you are sleeping right, there are high chances you are not getting enough sleep.

Do you experience low energy while working out?

Again, check your sleep time. Take a break from your workout routine for a couple of days, sleep well, and then get back to your workouts.

Do you feel tired in the evenings?

You may not be getting enough sleep.

Try a Power Nap

If you are someone who sleeps around 10:00 p.m. and wakes up at 5:30 a.m., then you may want to add this nap to your routine. It is a 15–20 minute nap; preferably post-lunch and it does offer benefits in terms of feeling fresh, just like what caffeine does to you. But do not exceed the time, as it can negate the benefits.

But I am at work, how can I power nap? (You too may have this question.)

Me: You do not need a bed (though great if you have it). Just close your eyes, stretch a bit on your chair, wear your eye mask and probably noise-cancelling headphones, and just relax. This will help. Initially, set an alarm on your cell to wake up.

Caution: this works well for many, but if you are someone who is an insomniac or cannot sleep at night, you should avoid power napping.

Chapter 21

Stress

Getting fit is an emotional journey full of rollercoaster rides!

How many agree with this?

Feeling happy and feeling sad are two of our main emotions that determine our mood. Both of them are linked to our expectations or expected results. When we get the expected results, we are happy and we feel good about what we do, whereas, when we don't get the expected results, we feel sad and we feel like quitting.

In the case of a fitness journey, our progress often moves up and down:

- There are some weeks where we get amazing results.

- And there are a few, where there is no progress at all or not as per our expectation. And this takes a toll on the emotional front.

Don't get stressed out on your fitness journey:

Ruby, an architecture student had started her fitness journey three weeks back. She was managing her meals well but was finding it difficult to beat her cravings for cookies.

Ruby: I have not eaten my favourite cookies for almost a month. And my sister keeps on eating it in front of me. You know how difficult it is for me to control myself!

Me: You know, eating it on a regular basis is not right for your fitness goal.

Ruby: I still controlled my craving, but this week, I have not dropped a single pound!

Me: I understand your frustration, but your journey is not limited to how many pounds you lose, we have discussed this, right?

Ruby: I understand that, but still, I am feeling sad.

This is not just Ruby's case, but many face these kinds of ups and downs and it leads to demotivation, causing enormous stress.

Why we should Manage Stress?

Stress can lead to poor eating habits which may result in fat gain.

E.g.: When you are stressed, you may forget to drink enough water or to sleep on time, which will impact your transformation journey.

Have you heard about emotional eating? Emotional eating is recognised as compulsive behaviour and is proof that your emotional state may affect how you eat. When you are stressed, there are high chances you may overeat or consume unhealthy foods or try some fad diets for quick results. The reason being, you are not in the right state of mind to put efforts to eat healthily. Whatever comes in front of you may find space in your stomach.

Stress causes mental fatigue and drains your energy too which can come in your way of exercising. It can also lead to headaches, chest pain, fatigue, high blood pressure, lack of focus, hormone imbalance, and reduced immunity.

Are Stress and Obesity linked? Of course, they are. Stress stimulates a series of brain signals and hormones that promote more eating of high fat/high sugar foods, which further stimulates over usage of insulin. Insulin promotes fat storage in fat cells, liver, and muscle leading to obesity.

STRESSED is DESSERTS spelt backwards!

Hence, stay away from desserts as far as possible 😊 and stay focused on your fitness journey.

How do we Manage It?

Manage your expectations! Avoiding stress is not always possible but identifying triggers and managing them can help.

Listing down a few tips:

Tip: Set your fitness goal objectively and keep your motivation high. *(We have already discussed a few techniques in one of the previous chapters.)*

Tip: Don't overlook non-scale parameters, as your journey is more than a math problem. We talk about holistic fitness and not just a number on a weighing scale.

Tip: Accept that even after making the best of plans and putting efforts, things can go wrong.

Tip: Connect with someone who is going through a similar journey. Sometimes, your family members or friends may not understand your frustration, but someone who is going through it can help you.

Tip: Practice 90 seconds of freeze. Look out for one good thing you achieved during the day and think about it for a minimum of 90 seconds. It can be the smallest of things like you were able to reach down to your kitchen cabinet and pick up the bag of grains on your own. Earlier you always needed your maid to lift it. Doing it will make you feel happy and you will do such things on a daily basis.

Tip: Control your negative self-talk. Feeling emotionally down can give rise to negative thoughts in your mind, which can absolutely spoil your journey if they are not controlled. Meditating for as little as five minutes a day has been found to be effective against it.

Tip: Rate your disturbing moments. Despite trying to stay positive, you may still get negative thoughts. So speak about it rather than suppressing them. You can also rate the discomfort they cause you on a scale of one to five. You may realise that they are not that destructive as they seem initially and can be managed.

Tip: Have your **Me-Time.** This method of stress reduction takes just a few minutes and can be done anywhere, you just need a quiet space.

- Close your eyes and think of a relaxing and pleasing image.

- Notice where your muscles are tight and relax them by taking a deep breath in through your nose to a count of four and then exhale slowly through your mouth to a count of eight.

- Notice how filling your whole body with air feels as you breathe in, and then notice the pause before you begin your exhale.

- Then relax and follow your natural breathing in and out for five minutes.

- Slowly loosen your attention and open your eyes.

This practice can calm your mind.

Tip: Celebrate your previous victories. Whenever you get good results, do you get an emotional high? The way you get low when you don't get results. If no, you are not celebrating your in-process victories.

Remember what I had mentioned about self-reward therapy and start doing it objectively.

And whenever you feel down, go back and remember your success stories and how you celebrated. It will not make you feel like a loser and enlighten your mood. Choose an enriching experience like a vacation rather than giving yourself some materialistic gifts for your in-process victories and it will give you the right boost to stay focused.

Tip: Stay consistent with your newfound lifestyle and give time to it.

Tip: Exercise is a great way to reduce stress. Include yoga, strength training, dancing, cycling, and running as a part of your routine. Exercise releases endorphins leading to a pleasure reaction and can help reduce stress.

Tip: Self-grooming helps. Taking self-care and keeping yourself groomed will help you look good and may not bother you much, especially on days you don't get expected results. It's not limited to shaving or waxing but wearing good clothes at home or while exercising. It will help you build good self-esteem.

Tip: Don't revolt, it's your own journey.

Tip: When you are constantly demotivated due to lack of results, there are chances you may revolt and go the other way round. What I mean is, sometimes the frustration levels go so high, that you will purposely eat junk or not follow a routine. Even though it might give you immediate satisfaction, you know that in the long run, it is sabotaging your journey.

Mera 50 gms bhi kam nahi hua pure hafte me, ab me kuch bhi follow nahi karunga. Abhi pizza aur pasta order karunga...... (I have not even lost 50 grams, hence I will not follow anything and resort to eating junk).

If this is what you get into, then you are in revolt mode. You may feel good till you eat, but then you know what happens when the guilt starts trickling in. So, stay away from such practices relax and get back to your routine as results may be just around the corner.

Tip: Most importantly, don't quit. *(Quitting might look like an easier option, but you will have to start over again.)*

Chapter 22
Child Obesity

Burgers are not for kids, said Vinay to his five-year-old, while munching on a jumbo burger at AFC.

But I need a small one, dada.

It will upset your stomach, let's have your favourite bread jam, said his dad as he cleaned his hands after finishing the burger.

What do you feel, his kid would think?

Khud kha raha hai, aur muzhe bata raha hai (He is eating a burger in front of his son and telling his son not to have it).

Our life as parents or elders is a live example for kids. They watch us closely and try to mimic us. We hardly see a fit parent having an overweight kid. (*Unless there is a medical condition.*) As fit parents focus on having the right lifestyle, they ensure they do the same with their kids.

But if you are the one having chips, cookies, chocolates, beverages at home, it is difficult to say no to your kids. You may still not give it to them, but since they have seen you have it, they will try consuming it in your absence.

We discussed not taking kids grocery shopping in one of the earlier chapters. Let's talk more about it:

Ron and Riya had planned a day-long shopping trip at a nearby mall on a weekend and their kid Rony got to know about it.

Rony: I want to come with you to the mall.

Mom: It's going to be a hectic day Rony, we have to shop for Diwali, you will get tired.

Rony: No, I will be all fine!

Mom: We have to get many things; you will get bored and then you will not allow us to shop.

Rony: Promise, I will not trouble you both.

Mom: Ok, then sleep early on Friday and we will leave at 9:00 a.m. on Saturday.

So, it's a Saturday morning, and Rony and his parents reach the mall at 10:00 a.m., hopefully with their shopping list ☺.

They shop for almost two hours with ease.

After two hours, Rony becomes restless.

Rony: Mom, I am hungry, I want French fries.

Mom: You had promised that you will behave like a good boy and not ask for junk food.

Rony: But I am hungry!

Mom: Let's see, when our shopping is done.

He keeps quiet for some time, and then again start nagging his mom.

Rony: Mom, please, I need it.

Now his dad becomes restless.

Dad: Ok, you can have it, but after that no more crying and troubling us.

Rony: Thank you, dada, you are so nice.

And they continue to shop and Rony enjoys the fries.

So, who should be blamed in the above scenario,

Rony or his dad? *I leave it to you to decide.*

The only reason his dad gave him the fries was so that he would allow them to shop peacefully. Not that one serving will immediately impact his health, but now Rony has liked the taste and there are high chances he will ask for more. Hence it is always better to avoid taking kids shopping. I know it will not be always feasible, but let's understand that child obesity is growing rapidly.

Golu – molu is no longer healthy!

Kids as young as two and three are suffering from health conditions like diabetes and a bad lifestyle is the primary reason behind it.

Who shows them this lifestyle? Kids don't eat this junk on their own. (At least for the first time). It is we who introduce them to such food items for whatever reasons, and they get used to it. And it's not just about food. If parents have become couch potatoes, then kids tend to copy them. Our kids see the world through us and if we become sedentary, then it is difficult to expect something different from them.

It does not just impact kids' physical health but also their social and emotional well-being, and self-esteem. It is also associated with poor academic performance and a lower quality of life.

There are various ways you can help your kid stay fit, but the best is to teach them about an active lifestyle. Don't just preach, practice it too, and lead by example.

Let's look at a few things which parents can focus on:

Tip: Restrict the usage of gadgets.

I know this is difficult, particularly in the COVID-19 era, where everything from school to coaching classes has turned digital. It is more important now as kids are getting a lot more screen time, so any additional screen time should be avoided at any cost. But if you keep the gadgets away, then you need to keep them engaged with some activities else, they may get bored.

Tip: Take kids to grounds/garden/play area

When I was a kid, I spent a lot of time playing outdoor sports and I'm sure most of you would have done the same because those were the only options available. I still remember, how my parents had to literally pull me away from the grounds and take me home. Now, we have to do the opposite, push kids out of the home and make them play some sport. And if it means that we need to play along with them, so be it. I am sure, once we do that and kids start generating interest, they will no longer be sedentary. And if history repeats itself, we may get the Saubhagya (fortune) of dragging them back home ☺.

Tip: Do not keep junk food at home

If you keep junk food at home, your kids will be tempted to try them and if they like the taste, they will consume it again and again. It's difficult to say no when that food item is already available in your kitchen. Hence be particular about what food you stock at home. Please read the nutrition labels and buy foods that will add value. Like I said earlier, kids will eat what we give them (*at least in the early years*), so it's our responsibility to feed them right.

If you are the one who stocks ice creams and beverages at home, then you can't stop your kids from eating them. You may still say no, but kids are smart enough to find their ways.

Tip: Have you heard of emotional bingeing?

Bad mood/lethargy and eating are related. People tend to end when they are emotionally down. The same is the case with kids. Our kids are often stressed due to academics which might lead to overeating. Keeping a healthy and peaceful environment at home will help the kids stay stress-free and will prevent them from overeating. The best thing a parent can give to their kid is their TIME.

Tip: Sleep on time

We have already seen the importance of sleeping on time and the same applies to kids who need more sleep. Sleep deprivation or late sleeping can irritate them and lead to overeating.

Avoiding late-night calls can be difficult due to work commitments but ensure that your kids are put to bed before you get on these calls.

Tip: Avoid taking them for grocery shopping (particularly in malls)

We are aware of the right shopping practices and why kids should not be taken along. One more point I want to highlight here is the impact of smart advertisements on kids. These ads are created with bright colours and promotional characters to attract the attention of children, and parents end up buying such junk food. Instead, take them to the local market or kirana (grocery) store and show them the raw materials used to make food. There are high chances that it might generate their interest to eat healthily.

While on a trip to Igatpuri's Manas resort, the owner of the resort, Nitin had gifted my son, Aaryan, a strawberry sapling and had told him to take care of it. When we got back home, Aaryan ensured that the plant was watered regularly, and it received the required sunlight as suggested. He observed it daily in anticipation of eating the first fruit and in the process, learnt how patient one has to be to enjoy the fruit. He could relate to the humungous efforts put in by our farmers and how important it is to not waste food. And when the first strawberry came, I can't describe how happy he was. I am sure if Nitin is reading this, he too will be very happy.

Tip: Educate your kids on good eating habits.

We have seen various aspects of fitness. Now, it's time to pass on the learnings to your family. Read one chapter along with them on a daily/weekly basis and I am sure they will learn the right things. Please note that obese kids are prone to get bullied in schools and colleges, which can impact their self-esteem a lot. Hence, ensure that you provide the required support to adopt healthy eating practices.

Tip: Teach them to cook meals

Kids like to learn new things, and this can be an interesting activity. When they get to know more about how food is cooked, what ingredients are used, they will learn more about nutrition, and how to eat the right foods. When you touch an apple, you feel the nutrition inside, whereas when you pick a burger, you will feel the junk inside (when you finish the burger). Similarly, kids can distinguish between good and bad foods when they are involved in the cooking process. Also, it can help them beat the hunger blues when they are alone at home/ hostel and they will not resort to ordering any junk.

Tip: Keep them in the company of grandparents as far as possible.

Grandparents teach valuable cultural lessons to kids through storytelling that kids find interesting. Right from village stories to eating habits to ancestral wisdom everything is discussed, which orient kids the right way. We talk a lot about getting back to our roots and there is no better way than having your kid learn such things from his/her nani-dadi.

Tip: Be your kid›s superhero

We all know the influence of superheroes on our little ones, but when we were kids, our favourite Popeye ate spinach. And unfortunately, Chota Bhim eats ladoos. So, it's our responsibility to be a superhero for our kids. No, I am not telling you to dress like one, unless it a fancy-dress competition! Be fit like a superhero and let your kid see the efforts you take to exercise, eat right and sleep on time.

Tip: Shouting and spanking will not help

You find out that your kid has finished a big burger, and you shout at him! This will not work in the long run. He may have seen you eating a burger and thus felt tempted to have one too.

Set the right example and kids will follow you.

Tip: Keep healthy eating challenges

Kids love challenges and they give their best participation. Create food-related challenges like drinking a glass of water every two hours or doing 30 jumping jacks for seven days in a row. Do reward them when they do that objectively.

Over and above these tips, do follow whatever we have discussed in the previous chapters and it will help in keeping your kid fit.

Chapter 23

What Next?

If you cannot run, then walk, and if you cannot walk then crawl …

Not sure where I read this, but I think this is so applicable to any fitness journey. It gives a simple message: **If you start taking action today it's amazing, don't wait for the perfect time.**

We have limitations and there are ways to tide over them. *(Chapter 2: Break The Barriers talks about it)*

"Can I overcome all of them instantly," asked Arun?

"Probably not, it will take some time," I replied.

"How much time?" he asked.

"The time starts once you begin implementing it."

"Hmmm…"

"See, it all lies in your head and you are waiting for some miracle to happen. Trust me, it doesn't work that way. You need to break those shackles and take the first step."

If you feel like exercising, do that.

If you think you can make an early dinner, start with that.

If you are keen on having more water, so be it.

If……

Today, you ask these questions as you have not taken the first step. And when you start, your questions will be:

How can I do better?

Can I get up early to find the time?

Should I drink warm water or normal water?

How…

Nothing changes our state of mind better than our efforts.

"Sounds good, I have a gym in my society, I will go there tomorrow," said Arun

"Wish you luck and do get back with your feedback," I told him.

I am sure Arun will work on his fitness. He may start exercising and will eventually focus on other aspects too. And why do I think he will do it? The simple answer is results. The slightest change in our body motivates us. I have seen people screaming with joy for losing just 50 grams and I am not exaggerating. I am sure some of you have had the same experiences. When Arun sees some tightness in his muscles, he will want to eat clean, sleep on time, drink enough water, etc. His interest will go up and eventually, he'll want to do everything.

That's what results can do…bring about a quick switch in our attitude. And a positive attitude compels you to take the required action.

Do it Now

Don't wait till next Monday or the new year or something else. So many Mondays have passed and I have seen most new year resolutions fading away in the first week of January itself.

Ask yourself, what was your best achievement to date, and recall how it all happened. It could be your academic results, or a complex project, or something else. Think about the **efforts** you put in to make the impossible look possible. Those **sleepless nights**, the **criticism** from your own people, the **initial failures**, and the way you **overcame** them all.

How do you feel now?

Isn't there a **blood rush?** (*kya romte khade ho gaye woh sab soch ke?*)

Do you feel like replicating that success?

Perfect, now look at your fitness goal and speak.

"I am going to conquer this too." Say it loudly, do not mind screaming it too.

And with this **positive attitude**, full of energy, **take your first step:**

Get up from your seat, take a **deep breath**, suck your stomach in and **START.**

Will the journey be easy?

May, or may not be. **But how does it matter?**

You have already won such battles in the past and this is for your own health and you will surely win.

LET'S GET GOING......... COME ON

Refer to this bird's eye view of all that we discussed:

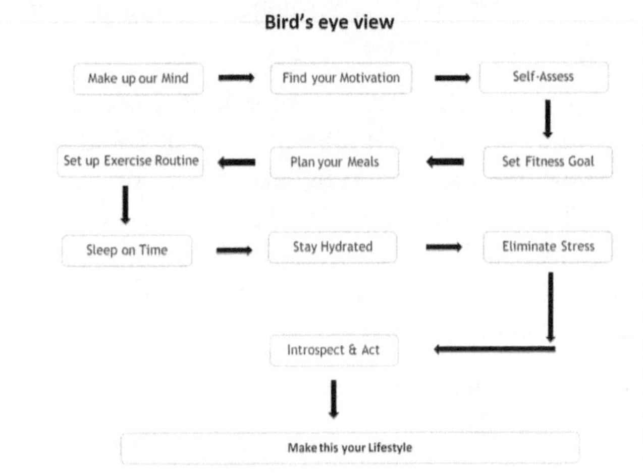

How Fitness Changed My Life: By Coach Anagha

Since my school days, I remember being active always and participating in sports events like gymnastics, swimming and table tennis. I also played sports at a competitive level. I was a state-level table tennis and district-level gymnastics player. However, it was a way for me to have fun and was never a serious career option.

Being active and playing sports as a hobby continued during my undergraduate college years. During my post-graduation years, the activity levels reduced with an increased focus on studies and the sudden seriousness of doing something for a career.

Securing a job in one of the top IT organisations as part of campus placements was one of the biggest successes at that point. However, in terms of health, this was the starting point of the deterioration of my health. An increase in work pressure, long work hours, a higher disposable income, and high-calorie food slowly influenced the body negatively. I gradually started piling on the weight. Like most professionals, I lost count of the number of teas and coffees I consumed daily at work.

Then, there was this beautiful phase of marriage and the post-marriage pampering. As I entered a new family, the lifestyle changes were many, including a shift from simple to rich, heavy food, more dinner outings, and increased socialisation. All this resulted in further weight gain.

Back pain, which had started during my office years, became aggravated. My increased weight added more pressure on my back. Being admitted at least once a year for rest and traction had become a routine. In fact, I was admitted four times in three years.

Then there was this phase of pregnancy. I had a healthy pregnancy, however, the post-pregnancy phase was a careless one, not just in terms of my eating habits, but also my bingeing and giving in to cravings. Under the guise of a baby and the additional responsibilities that come with it, I completely lost my health. I reached the peak of my weight gain during this period.

After a couple of years, I shifted from an IT organisation to a manufacturing company. A demanding, active toddler and an equally demanding career, the growing expectations of a new workplace and a different industry put my health in a bad state. It was not just the weight, which was scaling up, but the stress had gone up so much that on my return home from work I used to be breathless most of the time. The thing which hurt me the most was I was not able to lift my son and play with him. This bad health also made me highly impatient and I had low tolerance towards my son's demand for attention.

In the meantime, my husband had already increased his focus on fitness. He has been consistent in his fitness regime for the past 20 years and he was taking it to the next level by upping his skill in various forms like self-defence, personal training, and group coaching for a few office colleagues. Intermittently, I too joined him for about 1.5 years, participating in self-defence workshops. However, a bad back came in the way and I had to take frequent breaks and could not train too hard.

At that point, I decided to try one more time to get fit. The point to note is, this was not my first attempt to go on a weight loss journey. I tried multiple things earlier like going swimming, joining the gym not once but twice, going to a nutritionist, trying some fad, and crash diet. Some of these didn't help at all. While some gave temporary results but there was no consistency due to lack of time, motivation, commitments, etc.

However, this time, when I thought of doing something again, I knew that this was going to be my last attempt since I had already given up on myself.

"I am trying one more time," I told Bhushan.

"Let's work on it together," he replied. And my journey started.

This time, the focus was not just on weight loss, but a holistic health improvement and the method was not a typical diet and cardio but a beautiful combination of various things like eating right, exercising daily, sleeping on time, being active, etc. As my weight started shifting, my mindset also shifted from this being my last attempt to making it a part of my lifestyle. I realised and understood the importance of slow, sustainable, consistent weight loss. I also understood the importance of the parameters which are more important than mere body weight like muscle mass, low-fat percentage.

Multiple changes were happening for me from having a full meal dinner at 10:30 to having an early dinner and going to bed at 10:30. The initial one month of this journey was extremely frustrating, as efforts were put in but optimum results were not seen on the scale. That's when Bhushan made me realise that all changes cannot be measured on the scale. It may be intangible like a good night's sleep or when you have your proper monthly cycle. While getting up and doing the morning workouts was tough in the initial days, the feeling of freshness that I had for the entire day was good. I enjoyed being active, playing different sports with my son, lifting heavy weights, being able to have a good deep sleep, dressing up well, enjoying all the compliments and the likes on social media. I began enjoying good food and healthy options as well.

Looking at my health results, people around me started asking me about this concept and that's when I decided to get into wellness coaching with the primary intent of helping my friends and contacts. Time was always a challenge, however, the idea of passing on the benefits I had received to others was irresistible. I jumped into it and my journey as Wellness Coach Anagha started.

From then on, there was no looking back. Facilitating transformation as a wellness coach has been a very rewarding and satisfying experience. That 24 hours that each one of us gets seems to have doubled for me. It was really a big shift as initially, I struggled to get that half-hour for myself for my own workouts. But now, I spend about two to three hours with my participants and manage the rest with finesse. I understood it was all about *priorities in life. When your dreams and goals are big, the troubles automatically get underplayed.*

As a wellness coach, doing justice to your own work, managing time, managing investments, managing finances is not that easy, however with better clarity on goals it is possible.

My message to all those wanting to get fit, but are sitting on the fence:

"Jump in and have a fabulous journey, you deserve it."

Sharing my transformation pic to give you confidence that this works ☺.

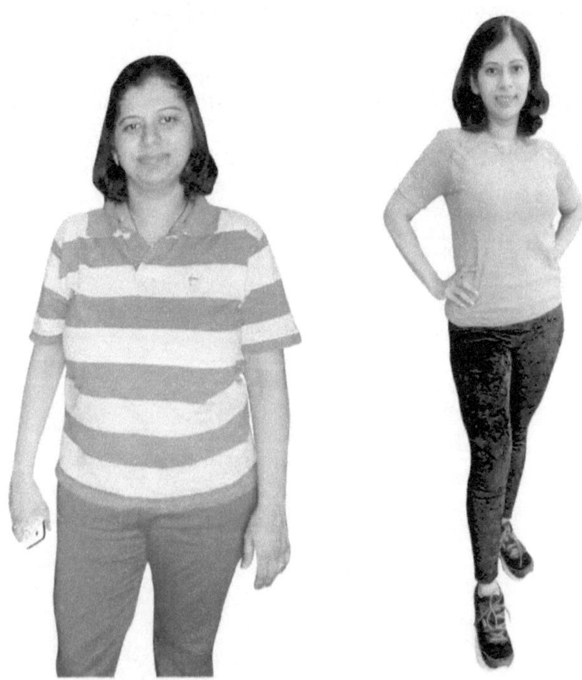

Transformation Story: Coach Anagha

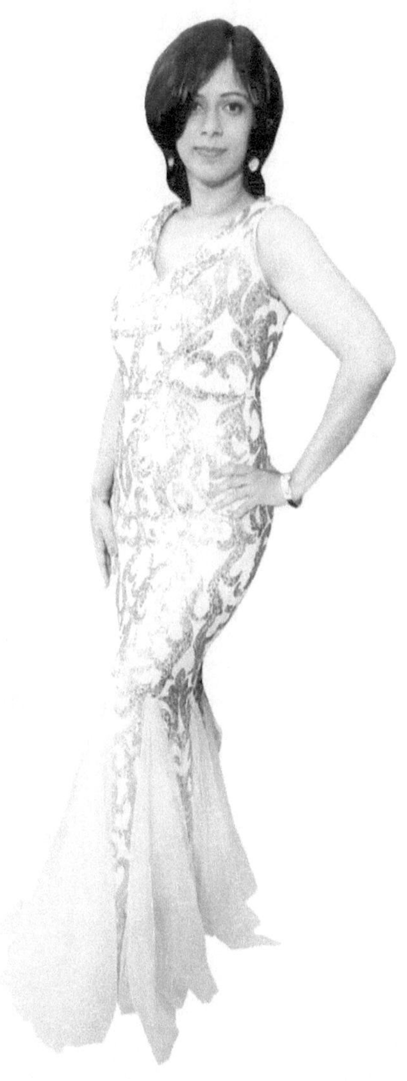

Transformation Story: Coach Anagha

Appendix and Resources

YouTube

I have created a YouTube channel that has a lot of videos on different aspects of fitness.

Please note these are unedited videos shot on a mobile phone. Please approach them with the intent of getting the required knowledge to initiate your fitness journey.

Link to my channel, Fitnessmessengers: https://youtube.com/channel/UCtJWvNNlra59Q7DITmMhUGA

It has the following videos:

- Warm-up and Cool-down exercise
- Upper Body workout
- Lower Body workout
- Full Body workout
- Core workout
- Beginner's core workout
- Partner's workout

- Workout using home props

- Muscle Mediation and many more

How to use these videos?

In the initial days, just focus on doing the warm-up and cool-down exercises and gradually add on to them. Learn techniques first and then look at adding more reps. Wherever you feel any pain or discomfort, take a break, and continue only when you are fine.

Social Media

Additionally, there are more resources on our Facebook and Instagram page: Fitnessmessengers.

Facebook: https://www.facebook.com/fitnessmessengers

Instagram: https://www.instagram.com/fitnessmessengers/

Fitnessmessengers Website

I have also created a website that can be used to plan your workouts. This is suitable for beginners and those who are pressed for time, as these exercises can be done in less than 20 minutes.

Our exercise videos are made in a way that it becomes feasible for anyone to follow them. Even those who have never exercised before can do it following the guidance provided. Gradually, the intensity of the exercise goes up as one progresses from one level to another.

We have laid down a road map that helps you move from Beginner to Intermediate to Expert over a span of time, thus building a strong foundation.

The process works as follows:

- We have created an exercise playlist for each day, and it has a warm-up sequence, followed by a functional session focused on a group of muscles, followed by a cool-down and stretching session.

- Each day the functional session varies depending on the group of muscles selected: Upper Body, Lower Body, Core, Full Body, etc.

- In each playlist, the exercises to be done are showcased along with the form and posture guidance.

Link to website: http://fitnessmessengers.com/

My Blogs

1. Too Busy to be Fit Now, will Wait for the Right Time

   https://fitnessmessengers.blogspot.com/2020/09/too-busy-to-be-fit-now-will-wait-for.html

2. I don't want anyone to know, I am working on my Fitness Goal.

   https://fitnessmessengers.blogspot.com/2020/09/i-dont-want-anyone-to-know-i-am-working.html

All the best for an amazing transformation. Make yourself Proud.

Acknowledgements

This book is conceptualised and written based on multiple Client Interactions, Group Discussions, Events, and Experiences. I would like to sincerely thank the following people because each one of them has made this book possible. This list is not exhaustive because naming every person is not possible.

So here goes.

- To my clients for sharing their routines, issues, their limitations, their failures. I could narrate their experiences as examples and make this book a relatable read. Multiple instances of clients from various backgrounds have adopted the Holistic Fitness way and have improved their lifestyle and this has strengthened my belief.

- To my corporate career, which helped me understand various constraints faced by other professionals leading to bad lifestyle. This exposure helped to coach empathetically and express the same in the book. Owing to space constraints, a large portion of the material from the interactions is not covered in this book. This material will have to wait for the next book.

- All my corporate colleagues and clients for looking up to me for fitness guidance. This gave me a boost to write about holistic fitness.

- To organisations and institutions for providing an opportunity to conduct Get Fit workshops and the Wellness Talks. This helped me consolidate my knowledge.

- All the fitness experts from whom I have got a deeper understanding of the various concepts.

- My Client and Society Acquaintance, Rajesh Saliya, for believing in Holistic Fitness and showcasing a healthy transformation and allowing me to share his story.

- To Ketaki Nagtilak, my colleague and now coach at Fitnessmessengers, for believing me in her transformation journey and sharing her thoughts.

- To Sangeeta Shetty for being a stress-buster friend and sharing her observations about the book's cover design.

- Rutika Kadam, my client as well as my illustrator, for translating my thoughts to beautiful sketches and enhancing the look of the book.

- My friends, Sandeep Bhadange and Dr Sanjyot Pethe, for giving me tips and taking me through the process of publishing a book.

- My publishing team at Notion Press: Rakesh, for patiently explaining the process and giving a physical form to my thoughts. Treesa for her candid feedback, Vignesh for introducing me to Notion Press and Mohammed for helping me throughout the process.

- My Aai for inculcating in me the right habits and choices in food from early stages in life, for teaching me the value of food, nutritionally and through traditional recipes. My parents may not believe the crazy ideas I work on but wholeheartedly supported me in everything.

- My wife, Anagha, for giving me space to work on the book, for taking home and other responsibilities and motivating me to write more. Also, for being the best critic for this book as well as supporting me with required examples and for all the rounds of getting my breakfast and water to our society terrace, the place where I wrote 90% of this book from 6-8 a.m.

- My eight-year-old son, Aaryan, for bearing with my absence every morning and declaring this book as the best book even when it was just half done.

- To my current team of coaches at Fitnessmesssngers: Sagar, Vinay, Ketaki, Artha, Anagha, Archana, Prita, Ujasvi, Narayan and Rutika for helping me spread the awareness of Holistic Fitness through our Online Fitness Programmes.

- I would also want to express my gratitude to the amazing place I had to write this book: the terrace of my building. The place has a vibe of its own and it really helped me write every single day.

- To Almighty for making me believe that I can write. ☺